Forever Young:

Mastering Intermittent Fasting for Women Over 50's Well-being

Manuel Carson

Table of Contents

Introduction

Welcome to "Forever Young"

Welcome to "Forever Young," where age is only a number and youth's spirit has no limitations. In our dynamic community, we believe that life is an adventure to be enjoyed to the fullest, regardless of age or circumstances. Whether you're a seasoned traveler on life's trip or just starting, "Forever Young" is your passport to a world of energy, pleasure, and limitless possibilities.

As we begin on this journey together, let us abandon the constraints of conventional knowledge in favor of a new paradigm of aging—one that values the wisdom of experience while embracing the energy of youth. Wrinkles are considered badges of distinction; laughing lines tell tales of joy and tenacity; and each gray hair is a monument to a life well lived.

In the next few pages, we'll look at the keys to keeping youthful in body, mind, and spirit. From promoting robust health and vitality to building a positive mentality and embracing new experiences, each chapter provides practical knowledge and actionable ideas to help you live your greatest life at any age.

So, whether you're looking for inspiration to rekindle your zest for life, advice on preserving physical and mental well-being, or just a community of like-minded people who refuse to let age define them, you've come to the perfect spot. Welcome to "Forever Young"—where the adventure never stops and the best is yet to come.

The Power of Intermittent Fasting

In recent years, intermittent fasting has been a fashionable health and wellness fad, with claims of multiple advantages ranging from weight reduction to enhanced metabolic health and lifespan. But what exactly is intermittent fasting, and why has it piqued the interest of so many individuals looking to improve their health and wellness?

In this part, we'll look at the science of intermittent fasting, including its origins, mechanics, and possible health advantages. From its ancient origins in religious and cultural rituals to its present comeback as a potent tool for health improvement, we'll reveal the mysteries of intermittent fasting and how it can change your life.

The Origins of Intermittent Fasting

Intermittent fasting is not a new concept; it has been used by societies all over the globe for millennia as a form of spiritual cleansing, ceremonial observance, and even as a technique for improving physical and mental performance. Fasting has played an important part in many cultures throughout history, from ancient religious traditions like Ramadan in Islam to the Christian custom of Lent.

Aside from its religious and cultural importance, intermittent fasting has been utilized for its alleged health advantages since ancient Greece, when luminaries such as Hippocrates, known as the founder of modern medicine, advised fasting as a treatment for a variety of diseases.

How Does Intermittent Fasting Work?

Intermittent fasting is essentially a cycle of eating and fasting to boost metabolic health, weight reduction, and lifespan. Intermittent fasting differs from standard calorie restriction diets in that it focuses on when you eat rather than what you consume.

Intermittent fasting may be accomplished by a variety of strategies, including:

1. Time-Restricted Eating: This entails restricting you're eating window to a certain time each day, such as an 8-hour window followed by a 16-hour fast.

2. Alternative-Day Fasting: This method entails alternating between days of regular eating and days of very low-calorie intake, or full fasting.

3. Periodic Fasting: Regularly, this entails fasting for significant durations, such as 24 hours or more.

Intermittent fasting, regardless of technique, promotes health and lifespan by activating the body's natural metabolic processes, such as ketosis and autophagy. During fasting, the body shifts from utilizing glucose as its major energy source to using fat reserves for fuel, resulting in weight reduction and better insulin sensitivity.

Health Benefits of Intermittent Fasting

Intermittent fasting has various demonstrated health advantages, including improved metabolic health, weight reduction, and lifespan. Some of the major advantages of intermittent fasting include:

1. Weight Loss: Intermittent fasting may help you lose weight and improve your body composition by lowering your calorie intake and increasing fat burning.

2. Improved Metabolic Health: Studies have indicated that intermittent fasting improves insulin sensitivity, reduces inflammation, and lowers the risk of chronic illnesses, including type 2 diabetes and heart disease.

3. Improved brain performance: Fasting has been associated with better cognitive performance, more attention, and a lower risk of neurodegenerative disorders, including Alzheimer's and Parkinson's.

4. Longevity: Animal studies have indicated that intermittent fasting may lengthen lifespan and postpone the development of

age-related disorders, raising the possibility that it will have comparable benefits in humans.

Getting Started with Intermittent Fasting

If you want to use intermittent fasting to enhance your health and well-being, getting started is simpler than you would imagine. Begin by choosing an intermittent fasting approach that fits your lifestyle and objectives, and then progressively increase your fasting window over time.

To maintain optimum health and energy levels, emphasize nutrient-dense meals during feeding times and keep hydrated during the fasting phase. Remember that intermittent fasting is not a one-size-fits-all strategy; experimentation and personalization are essential for discovering the fasting schedule that works best for you.

In the following chapters, we'll go over the various techniques of intermittent fasting in greater depth, delving deeper into the science behind its possible health advantages, and providing practical suggestions and tactics for incorporating intermittent fasting into your daily routine. So saddle up and prepare to embark on a journey of improved health, energy, and longevity with the power of intermittent fasting.

Why Intermittent Fasting Is Important for Women Over 50

As women age, maintaining good health becomes more critical for their general well-being and energy. Women over 50 have distinct problems as they age, ranging from hormonal changes to metabolic adjustments. However, intermittent fasting has emerged as a strong tool for assisting women in navigating these changes and optimizing their health in their older years. In this part, we'll look at why intermittent fasting is important for women over 50, including possible advantages, concerns, and practical application tactics.

Recognizing Women Over 50's Unique Health Challenges

Before delving into the mechanics of intermittent fasting, it's critical to understand the distinct health issues that women over 50 may encounter. As women go through menopause and beyond, they may encounter several physical and hormonal changes that affect their health and well-being. This may include:

1. Hormonal Changes: The decrease in estrogen levels during menopause may cause changes in metabolism, bone density, and body composition.

2. Weight Management: Many women find it increasingly difficult to maintain a healthy weight as they age, owing to metabolic changes and hormonal swings.

3. Bone Health: Lower estrogen levels may raise the risk of osteoporosis and bone fractures in postmenopausal women.

4. Heart Health: Women over 50 are more likely to develop heart disease, especially after menopause, owing to increases in cholesterol and blood pressure.

Given these limitations, finding effective measures to promote optimum health and well-being becomes critical for women over 50. Intermittent fasting may be a potential strategy.

Benefits of Intermittent Fasting for Women Over 50

Intermittent fasting has been found to have several advantages, especially for women over the age of 50. This includes:

1. Weight Management: Intermittent fasting may help women over 50 maintain a healthy weight by increasing fat loss, improving insulin sensitivity, and lowering the risk of age-related weight gain.

2. Metabolic Health: Studies have indicated that fasting improves metabolic health indicators such as blood sugar levels, cholesterol levels, and blood pressure, all of which are crucial in avoiding chronic illnesses, including type 2 diabetes and heart disease.

3. Hormonal Balance: According to some studies, intermittent fasting may help control hormone levels in women, such as estrogen and insulin, which may benefit general health and well-being.

4. Brain Health: Fasting has been linked to enhanced cognitive function, memory, and mood, which may be especially advantageous for women over the age of 50, who are at higher risk for cognitive decline.

Considerations for Women Over 50

While intermittent fasting may provide several advantages for women over the age of 50, it is essential to proceed with care and consider personal health requirements and circumstances. Some essential concerns are:

1. Hormonal Changes: Women going through menopause or perimenopause may have specific hormonal factors that influence their response to intermittent fasting. Before beginning any fasting program, contact a healthcare practitioner, particularly if you have hormone imbalances or other underlying health concerns.

2. Bone Health: Women over 50 are more likely to develop osteoporosis and bone fractures, so it's important to get enough calcium and vitamin D and add weight-bearing workouts to your regimen to promote bone health.

3. Nutritional needs: As we get older, our nutritional demands may alter, so it's vital to consume nutrient-dense meals and get enough protein to sustain muscle mass and general health.

Effective Strategies for Implementing Intermittent Fasting

If you're a woman over 50 who wants to practice intermittent fasting, here are some practical techniques to get started:

1. Begin Slowly: If you're new to intermittent fasting, gradually extend the duration of your fasting window over time to enable your body to acclimate.

2. Choose the appropriate method: There are various techniques of intermittent fasting, so choose one that fits your lifestyle and objectives. Popular choices include time-restricted eating, alternate-day fasting, and intermittent fasting.

3. Keep Hydrated: When fasting, drink lots of water to keep hydrated and promote general health and well-being.

4. Listen to Your Body: Monitor how your body reacts to intermittent fasting and alter your strategy as required. If you encounter any unpleasant side effects or discomfort, you should reconsider your fasting regimen or seek advice from a healthcare practitioner.

Conclusions:

Intermittent fasting has enormous promise as a strong strategy for improving the health and well-being of women over 50. By encouraging weight control, metabolic health, hormonal balance, and brain health, intermittent fasting may help women traverse the specific difficulties of aging with grace and energy. However, intermittent fasting should be approached with prudence, considering individual health demands and circumstances. With the correct strategy and supervision, intermittent fasting may be a beneficial supplement to a healthy lifestyle for women over 50, allowing them to enjoy life to the fullest for years to come.

Chapter 1: The Science Behind Intermittent Fasting

Exploring the Physiology of Aging

Welcome to Chapter 1 of our exploration of the science of intermittent fasting and its enormous implications for the aging process. In this chapter, we'll look at the physiology of aging, including the complex pathways that cause cellular decline, metabolic dysfunction, and age-related disorders. Understanding the basic mechanisms of aging allows us to better understand how intermittent fasting counteracts these impacts while increasing health, energy, and longevity.

The Aging Process: A Biological View

Aging is a complicated and diverse process that affects every cell, tissue, and organ in our bodies. While the precise mechanics of aging are still not completely understood, scientists have found many essential markers that describe the aging process:

1. Genomic Instability: As time passes, DNA damage accumulates in cells, causing mutations and genomic instability, which may contribute to cellular malfunction and aging.

2. Telomere Shortening: As cells divide, telomeres, the protective caps at the ends of chromosomes, shorten, ultimately contributing to cellular senescence and aging.

3. Epigenetic Alterations: As people age, their gene expression patterns change, affecting cellular function and contributing to age-related disorders.

4. Proteostasis Loss: As we age, the body's capacity to maintain protein homeostasis, also known as proteostasis, weakens, resulting in the buildup of misfolded proteins and cellular malfunction.

5. Mitochondrial Dysfunction: As cells age, mitochondria, which are the energy-producing organelles inside them, lose efficiency, resulting in reduced energy generation and oxidative stress.

6. Cellular Senescence: As cells age, they reach a condition called senescence, in which they stop dividing and contribute to tissue malfunction and inflammation.

7. Stem Cell Exhaustion: As stem cells age, their regenerative ability reduces, resulting in decreased tissue repair and regeneration.

The Role of Metabolism in Aging

Metabolism is crucial to the aging process, impacting cellular function, energy generation, and general health. As we get older, our metabolic function becomes less effective, resulting in abnormalities in energy homeostasis, nutrition sensing, and mitochondrial function. These metabolic alterations are linked to age-related illnesses such as obesity, type 2 diabetes, cardiovascular disease, and neurodegenerative disorders.

How Intermittent Fasting Affects Aging Physiology

Intermittent fasting has a significant impact on aging physiology, affecting various pathways involved in age-related decline and illness. Intermittent fasting alters aging physiology in many important ways, including:

1. Enhanced Autophagy: Fasting promotes autophagy, a cellular process that eliminates damaged organelles and proteins, resulting in cell rejuvenation and longevity.

2. Improved Metabolic Health: Fasting increases insulin sensitivity, decreases inflammation, and stimulates fat burning, resulting in better metabolic health and a decreased risk of age-related disorders.

3. Increased Mitochondrial Biogenesis: Fasting promotes the formation of new mitochondria, increasing cellular energy output while decreasing oxidative stress.

4. Fasting promotes sirtuins, a protein family that regulates cellular metabolism, DNA repair, and lifespan.

5. Reduction in Oxidative Stress: Fasting lowers oxidative stress and inflammation, protecting cells and increasing lifespan.

6. Enhanced Stem Cell Function: Fasting increases stem cells' regenerative potential, boosting tissue repair and regeneration.

Practical Considerations for Implementing Intermittent Fasting:

While the research underpinning intermittent fasting is convincing, it is critical to proceed with care and account for individual health requirements and circumstances. Here are some practical concerns for practicing intermittent fasting:

1. Start Slowly: If you're new to fasting, gradually extend the duration of your fasting window over time to enable your body to acclimate.

2. Keep Hydrated: When fasting, drink lots of water to stay hydrated and promote overall health and well-being.

3. Listen to Your Body: Pay attention to how your body reacts to fasting and alter your strategy as necessary. If you encounter any unpleasant side effects or discomfort, you should reconsider your fasting regimen or seek advice from a healthcare practitioner.

Conclusions:

In this chapter, we looked at the complicated physiology of aging and how intermittent fasting may help prevent age-related decline and illness. Intermittent fasting has enormous potential as a strong tool for boosting health, vitality, and longevity since it targets critical aging mechanisms such as autophagy, metabolism, and mitochondrial function. However, fasting should be approached with prudence, considering individual health demands and circumstances. In the next chapters, we'll go further into the science of intermittent fasting, investigating its impact on certain elements of health and aging, and offering practical advice and tactics for integrating fasting into your daily routine.

How It Affects Aging Processes

Welcome to Chapter 1 of our investigation into the science of intermittent fasting (IF) and its dramatic impact on aging processes. In this chapter, we'll look at the complicated processes that support the IF-aging link. From cellular rejuvenation to metabolic optimization, IF has emerged as a viable method for improving health and lifespan. By delving into scientific studies, we may discover how IF affects aging at the molecular, cellular, and systemic levels, paving the way for a better understanding of its transforming potential.

Exploring the Biology of Aging:

Aging is a complex phenomenon marked by a steady reduction in physiological performance and an increasing vulnerability to illness. While aging is impacted by a plethora of variables, including genetics, lifestyle, and environmental exposures, five major mechanisms govern its progression:

1. Cellular Senescence: Senescence is a process in which aging cells stop dividing and amass over time. Senescent cells generate pro-inflammatory chemicals, which lead to tissue dysfunction and aging-related diseases.

2. Oxidative Stress: As we age, the balance of oxidants and antioxidants in our bodies shifts, resulting in increased oxidative stress. This oxidative damage may impede cellular function and accelerate the aging process.

3. Mitochondrial Dysfunction: The mitochondria, the cell's powerhouse, endure age-related reductions in function and efficiency. Reduced mitochondrial activity may hinder cellular energy generation while increasing oxidative stress.

4. Inflammation: Chronic low-grade inflammation, also known as inflammation, is a sign of aging and leads to the development of age-related disorders such as cardiovascular disease, Alzheimer's disease, and cancer.

5. Genomic Instability: As cells age, they accumulate DNA damage and mutations, which causes genomic instability and increases the risk of cancer and other age-related illnesses.

Effects of Intermittent Fasting on Aging Processes:

Intermittent fasting has emerged as a powerful strategy for slowing aging and increasing health. IF has a significant impact on aging at many levels because of its effects on metabolism, cellular signaling, and stress response pathways.

1. Autophagy Activation: Intermittent fasting stimulates autophagy, a cellular mechanism that removes damaged organelles and proteins to aid in cellular repair and rejuvenation. Autophagy is crucial for maintaining cellular homeostasis and preventing age-related deterioration.

2. Metabolic Optimization: Fasting causes metabolic alterations that increase insulin sensitivity, mitochondrial function, and fat utilization. These metabolic adjustments help to improve general health and may prevent the emergence of age-related metabolic diseases, including type 2 diabetes and obesity.

3. Reduction of Inflammation: IF has anti-inflammatory properties, inhibiting the generation of pro-inflammatory cytokines and reducing chronic low-grade inflammation. By suppressing inflammatory signaling pathways, fasting may lower the risk of age-related inflammatory disorders.

4. Increased Stress Resistance: Fasting stimulates cellular stress response pathways, such as the sirtuin and AMPK pathways, which aid cells in adapting to and surviving external stresses. These

pathways boost cellular resilience and may help protect against age-related damage.

5. DNA repair and longevity: Studies have demonstrated that intermittent fasting improves DNA repair processes, lowering the buildup of DNA damage and mutations linked to aging. Fasting may improve longevity by preserving genomic integrity and delaying the development of age-related illnesses.

Practical Considerations for Intermittent Fasting:

While the scientific data supporting the health advantages of intermittent fasting is substantial, fasting should be approached with awareness and regard for individual needs and circumstances.

1. Personalization: There is no one-size-fits-all method for intermittent fasting. Experiment with various fasting procedures to see what works best for your body and lifestyle.

2. Nutrient Density: Consume nutrient-dense meals during eating windows to ensure your body gets enough vitamins, minerals, and macronutrients.

3. Hydration: To stay hydrated during fasting times, consume lots of water, herbal tea, and other non-caloric liquids.

4. Monitor Symptoms: Pay attention to your body's reaction to fasting and change your strategy appropriately. If you encounter unfavorable side effects such as weariness, dizziness, or irritability, you should reconsider your fasting schedule or visit a healthcare expert.

Conclusions:

In this chapter, we investigated the complex interaction between intermittent fasting and aging processes, revealing how fasting affects cellular function, metabolism, and lifespan. Intermittent fasting has the potential to be a revolutionary strategy for increasing life expectancy and enhancing vitality in the elderly by leveraging the power of autophagy, metabolic optimization, and stress tolerance. In the next chapters, we'll look further into the scientific data supporting intermittent fasting and its impact on particular age-related illnesses, as well as provide practical insights and advice for integrating fasting into your daily routine.

Advantages of Intermittent Fasting for Women Over 50

Welcome to Chapter 1 of our investigation into the science of intermittent fasting (IF) and its specific advantages for women over 50. In this chapter, we'll look at the physiological and metabolic changes that occur with aging, as well as how intermittent fasting may be an effective technique for maintaining health and longevity in women at this stage of life. From hormonal balance to cognitive function, IF provides a slew of advantages that may help women over 50 stay healthy and flourish as they age.

Understanding the aging process in women:

As women approach their fifth decade and beyond, they experience several hormonal and metabolic changes that might affect their health and well-being.

1. Hormonal Shifts: Menopause is the end of reproductive function and is characterized by a decrease in estrogen and progesterone levels. These hormonal fluctuations might cause symptoms including hot flashes, mood swings, and sleep difficulties.

2. Metabolic Changes: As people age, their metabolic rate, muscle mass, and bone density decrease, while visceral fat storage increases. These alterations may raise the risk of weight gain, insulin resistance, and chronic conditions including heart disease and osteoporosis.

3. Cognitive Decline: As people age, their cognitive function declines, including memory, attention, and executive function. Hormonal oscillations and metabolic alterations may also contribute to cognitive deterioration in women over 50.

Benefits of Intermittent Fasting for Women Over 50:

Intermittent fasting has a variety of advantages that may help women over 50 maintain their health and vigor as they age.

1. Weight Management: Intermittent fasting may help women over 50 lose fat, maintain lean muscle mass, and improve metabolic health. Fasting may help you lose weight by lowering your calorie intake and improving fat oxidation.

2. Hormonal Balance: Intermittent fasting has been proven to promote hormonal balance in women by reducing insulin resistance, decreasing insulin and leptin levels, and improving sensitivity to sex hormones like estrogen and progesterone. These hormonal changes may help reduce menopausal symptoms while also improving overall health.

3. Metabolic Health: Fasting offers metabolic advantages that may assist women over 50 in maintaining good health. Fasting may help prevent and control metabolic disorders, including type 2 diabetes, cardiovascular disease, and metabolic syndrome, by increasing insulin sensitivity, lowering inflammation, and encouraging cellular repair and regeneration.

4. Cognitive performance: A new study indicates that intermittent fasting may have neuroprotective benefits and improve cognitive performance in women over 50. Fasting may help maintain cognitive function and lower the risk of age-related neurodegenerative disorders such as Alzheimer's disease by lowering oxidative stress, increasing the production of brain-derived neurotrophic factor (BDNF), and encouraging the creation of new neurons.

5. Lifespan: Intermittent fasting has been related to enhanced lifespan and health in animal studies, and it may have comparable effects in humans. Fasting may help women over 50 live longer,

healthier lives by boosting cellular repair processes, lowering inflammation, and increasing metabolic health.

Practical Considerations for Intermittent Fasting:

While intermittent fasting may provide several advantages for women over 50, it is essential to proceed with care and take into account individual health requirements and circumstances.

1. Begin Slowly: If you're new to intermittent fasting, start with shorter fasts and gradually increase the length as your body adjusts.

2. Keep Hydrated: While fasting, drink lots of water to keep hydrated and maintain cellular activity.

3. Listen to Your Body: Pay attention to how your body reacts to fasting, and adjust your strategy accordingly. If you suffer any undesirable side effects, such as weariness or lightheadedness, reconsider your fasting routine or seek advice from a healthcare practitioner.

4. Combine with a Healthy Lifestyle: Intermittent fasting works best when accompanied by a nutritious diet, regular physical exercise, enough sleep, and stress management techniques.

Conclusions:

In this chapter, we looked at the science underlying intermittent fasting and its specific advantages for women over 50. From hormonal balance to metabolic health, cognitive function, and lifespan, IF provides a variety of benefits that may help women face the difficulties of aging with grace and energy. In the following chapters, we'll go over the practical components of intermittent fasting, including advice, methods, and meal plans to help women over 50 adopt fasting into their everyday lives and enjoy the benefits of this powerful health tool.

Chapter 2: Preparing for Your Intermittent Fasting Journey

Assessing Your Current Lifestyle and Diet

Welcome to Chapter 2 of your intermittent fasting experience! Before starting any new health routine, you should assess your present lifestyle and eating habits. In this chapter, we'll walk you through a thorough evaluation of your daily routines, eating habits, and general health to lay the groundwork for a successful intermittent fasting journey. Gaining a greater awareness of your abilities, problems, and objectives will allow you to personalize your fasting strategy to your requirements and preferences.

Evaluate Your Current Lifestyle:

Reflect on your present lifestyle and identify areas where you may need to make changes to assist your intermittent fasting journey.

1. Sleep Patterns: Evaluate your sleep patterns, such as bedtime rituals, sleep length, and quality. Aim for 7-9 hours of undisturbed sleep every night to promote overall health and well-being.

2. Physical Activity: Assess your workout regimen to see whether you're getting enough physical activity to meet your objectives. To increase total health and vitality, combine aerobic activity with strength training and flexibility activities.

3. Stress Management: Consider how you handle stress in your everyday life and devise techniques to reduce stress levels. Incorporate stress-relieving hobbies such as meditation, yoga, deep breathing exercises, or spending time outside.

4. Social Support: Consider your social relationships and support groups. Surround yourself with friends, family, and community members who will support and encourage you on your health path.

5. Work-Life Balance: Evaluate your work-life balance and aim to establish clear boundaries between work and personal time. Prioritize activities that provide you with pleasure and contentment outside of work.

Assessing Your Current Diet:

Next, let's look at your present food patterns and find places for improvement.

1. Eating Patterns: Assess your regular eating habits, such as meal schedule, frequency, and portion size. Are you eating balanced meals at regular intervals throughout the day, or do you skip meals and graze mindlessly?

2. Nutritional Intake: Evaluate the nutritional quality of your food to see whether it meets your body's requirements for important vitamins, minerals, and macronutrients. Include a variety of nutrient-dense foods in your meals, such as fruits and vegetables, whole grains, lean meats, and healthy fats.

3. Hydration: Monitor your fluid intake to ensure you're staying hydrated throughout the day. Aim for at least 8–10 glasses of water every day and restrict your intake of sugary and caffeinated beverages.

4. Mindful Eating: Consider your connection to food and how you approach eating. When eating, pay attention to hunger and fullness signals, appreciate each mouthful, and minimize distractions like computers or electronic gadgets.

5. Food Choices: Examine the types of meals you usually eat and identify any areas where you may need to make changes. Reduce

your intake of processed meals, sugary snacks, and harmful fats, and instead fuel your body with whole, minimally processed foods.

Goals for Your Intermittent Fasting Journey:

Now that you've evaluated your existing lifestyle and nutrition, select precise, attainable objectives for your intermittent fasting journey:

1. Define Your Why: Explain why you are starting this path and what you want to achieve. Having a strong sense of purpose can help you stay motivated and focused on your objectives, whether they be to improve your health, increase your energy, or lose weight.

2. Set SMART Goals: Create SMART (specific, measurable, achievable, relevant, and time-bound) goals that are consistent with your overall objectives. Break down huge objectives into smaller, more manageable stages, and measure your progress along the way.

3. Identify any difficulties: Prepare for any hurdles or difficulties that may occur throughout your fasting journey and devise solutions to overcome them. Having a plan in place can help you remain on track while dealing with hunger cravings, navigating social settings, or adapting to new eating habits.

4. Seek Support: Enlist the aid of friends, family, or a health coach to keep you accountable and motivated throughout your intermittent fasting journey. Share your objectives and accomplishments with others who can provide support and direction along the way.

5. Celebrate Progress: Acknowledge your accomplishments and milestones along the road, no matter how tiny. Recognize and celebrate your accomplishments, and utilize each one as fuel to move you ahead on your path to maximum health and well-being.

Conclusions:

In this chapter, we discussed the significance of evaluating your existing lifestyle and nutrition patterns as you prepare for your intermittent fasting adventure. By assessing your daily routines, eating habits, and general health, you'll obtain vital information that will allow you to personalize your fasting strategy to your specific requirements and objectives. With a better awareness of your talents, problems, and goals, you're ready to go on this revolutionary health path with confidence and purpose. In the next chapters, we'll go over the practical components of intermittent fasting, including advice, methods, and meal plans to help you succeed on your journey to better health and energy.

Setting Realistic Wellness and Longevity Goals

Welcome to Chapter 2 of your intermittent fasting experience! In this chapter, we'll look at how important it is to create realistic objectives for your health and longevity as you begin on this revolutionary path. Establishing defined targets and milestones will better prepare you to manage the obstacles and possibilities that lie ahead, resulting in long-term success in improving your health and well-being through intermittent fasting.

Understanding Goal Setting's Importance

Setting objectives is an essential stage in any path of personal development and self-improvement. Goals give direction, concentration, and incentive, allowing you to remain on track and assess your progress along the way. When it comes to intermittent fasting, creating realistic and attainable objectives is critical for long-term success and sustainability.

1.   Clarity: Define   your   aims   clearly and specifically. Determine what you want to accomplish with intermittent fasting, whether it's weight reduction, better

metabolic health, greater cognitive function, or an extended lifespan.

2. Measurability: Make sure your objectives are measurable and quantifiable. Set success metrics or criteria that can be tracked and evaluated over time. Factors such as body weight, body composition, blood sugar, cholesterol, cognitive function, and overall quality of life may be included.

3. Achievability: Set objectives that are demanding yet reachable. When making objectives, take into account your present health, lifestyle choices, and personal situations, and strive for improvement rather than perfection. Break down huge objectives into smaller, more manageable stages to make them more attainable.

4. Relevance: Make your objectives consistent with your beliefs, priorities, and ambitions. Select objectives that are personally important and relevant to your overall health and quality of life. Consider how reaching these objectives will benefit many elements of your life, such as physical health and mental well-being, relationships, and personal satisfaction.

5. Time-bound: Set a schedule or deadline for completing your objectives to instill urgency and responsibility. Set short-term, medium-term, and long-term objectives with deadlines for fulfillment. Regularly evaluate and update your objectives to ensure they are still relevant and attainable as you continue through your intermittent fasting adventure.

Setting realistic goals for health and longevity:

Now, let's look at three major areas where you may establish realistic objectives for increasing your health, well-being, and longevity via intermittent fasting:

1. Weight Management: If weight reduction is one of your key objectives, establish realistic targets for how much weight you want to lose over a specific period. Aim for a steady, sustained weight reduction of 1-2 pounds each week, which is both feasible and beneficial in the long run.

2. Metabolic Health: Set targets to improve important metabolic health indicators such as blood sugar, insulin sensitivity, and cholesterol. Intermittent fasting and healthy lifestyle modifications may help you decrease fasting blood sugar levels, reduce insulin resistance, and enhance lipid profiles.

3. Cognitive Function: Set objectives to improve cognitive function and brain health via intermittent fasting. Over time, measure gains in cognitive performance, memory, attention, and mental clarity, as well as changes in brain health indicators such as brain-derived neurotrophic factor (BDNF) levels.

4. Physical Fitness: If physical fitness is a top objective, create goals for developing strength, endurance, flexibility, and general fitness. Objective measurements of improvement include strength growth, cardiorespiratory fitness tests, flexibility examinations, and body composition studies.

5. Longevity: Set objectives to promote longevity and good aging via intermittent fasting. Aim to minimize inflammation, oxidative stress, and other aging indicators while increasing cellular repair, regeneration, and resilience. Assess your progress towards longevity goals by measuring improvements in biological age, telomere length, and other aging indicators.

Practical Tips for Achieving Your Goals:

As you establish and pursue your health and longevity objectives via intermittent fasting, consider the following practical recommendations to improve your chances of success:

1. Be consistent. Maintaining consistency is essential for attaining your intermittent fasting objectives. To get the most benefits from fasting, stick to your fasting schedule, diet plan, and lifestyle habits regularly.

2. Track Your Progress: Use a notebook, smartphone app, or other monitoring tools to monitor your progress toward your objectives. To stay informed and motivated, track critical indicators, milestones, and changes in health factors.

3. Celebrate triumphs: Recognize your triumphs and accomplishments along the path, no matter how minor. Recognize and reward yourself for reaching milestones and moving toward your objectives.

4. Be Flexible: Be willing to adapt your objectives and techniques as required based on input from your body, changes in circumstances, or new knowledge. Maintain adaptability and flexibility in your approach to intermittent fasting and goal-setting.

5. Seek Support: Don't be afraid to seek help from friends, family members, or healthcare experts while you work toward your objectives. Share your objectives with people who can provide support, accountability, and assistance along the way.

Conclusions:

In this chapter, we discussed the necessity of establishing realistic health and lifespan objectives as you begin your intermittent fasting journey. By defining specific targets, setting measurable milestones, and remaining focused on your priorities, you'll be better able to achieve long-term success in improving your health, well-being, and quality of life through intermittent fasting. In the next chapters, we'll go over the practical components of intermittent fasting, including advice, methods, and meal plans to help you reach your objectives and realize the full potential of this revolutionary health tool.

Creating a Customized Intermittent Fasting Plan

Introduction:

Welcome to Chapter 2 of your intermittent fasting experience! In this chapter, we'll walk you through the process of designing a customized intermittent fasting strategy that is tailored to your requirements, tastes, and lifestyle. By adapting your fasting strategy to your specific needs, you can maximize the advantages of intermittent fasting while reducing any obstacles or negatives. Whether you're new to fasting or have some experience, this chapter will guide you through the process of creating a plan that will set you up for success on your path to better health and wellness.

Understanding Intermittent Fasting:

Before we get into the mechanics of establishing your fasting schedule, let's go over the fundamentals of intermittent fasting and how it works:

1. Definition: Intermittent fasting is a dietary plan that alternates between periods of fasting and eating. Unlike typical diets, which concentrate on what you eat, intermittent fasting focuses on when you eat, to improve metabolic health, weight reduction, and general well-being.

2. Fasting programs: You may pick from a variety of intermittent fasting programs, including:

Time-Restricted Eating: This strategy entails restricting your eating window to a specified time each day, usually 8–12 hours, with the other hours set aside for fasting.

Alternate-Day Fasting: This strategy entails alternating between days of regular eating and days of fasting, either by ingesting extremely few calories or abstaining from food altogether.

5:2 Diet: Under this strategy, you eat normally five days a week and limit your calorie intake to 500–600 calories on two non-consecutive days.

Periodic Fasting: Regularly, this method entails fasting for prolonged durations, such as 24 hours or more, which might range from once or twice a week to once a month.

3. Health Benefits: Intermittent fasting has been demonstrated to improve metabolic health, promote weight reduction, raise insulin sensitivity, decrease inflammation, and improve cognitive function. It may also improve longevity by promoting cellular repair and regeneration.

Assessing Your Goals and Preferences:

Before developing an intermittent fasting strategy, consider your objectives, preferences, and lifestyle factors:

1. Health Goals: Explain why you're trying intermittent fasting and what you expect to accomplish. Whether your objectives are weight reduction, improved metabolic health, greater energy levels, or general well-being, having a strong sense of purpose can help you navigate your fasting path.

2. own tastes: Before deciding on a fasting plan, consider your tastes and lifestyle. Consider your job schedule, family responsibilities, social activities, and exercise regimen before choosing a plan that meets your requirements and preferences.

3. Past Experience: Consider any previous fasting or dietary changes. Consider what has worked successfully for you in the past, as well as any issues you have had, and use this knowledge to guide your approach to intermittent fasting.

Designing Your Fasting Plan:

Now that you understand intermittent fasting as well as your individual goals and preferences, it's time to create your fasting plan.

1. Choose a Fasting Protocol: Choose the intermittent fasting protocol that is most appropriate for your objectives, interests, and lifestyle. Experiment with many methods until you find one that seems sustainable and enjoyable to you.

2. Determine Your Eating Window: Choose the length of your eating window, which will determine when you eat your meals and

snacks. Aim for a timeframe that enables you to achieve your dietary requirements while still offering enough fasting time for maximum health advantages.

3. Establish fasting and feeding times: Depending on your protocol, specify when you will begin and conclude your fasting and feeding intervals each day or week. Consistency is essential, so try to adhere to your scheduled times as precisely as possible.

4. Plan Your Meals: After you've determined your eating window, schedule your meals and snacks appropriately. To promote your health and well-being, eat nutrient-dense, whole meals that include a balanced combination of macronutrients and micronutrients.

5. Hydration and supplementation: To keep hydrated throughout your fasting times, consume lots of water, herbal tea, or other calorie-free liquids. Consider adding electrolytes or other supplements as required to help you fast and stay hydrated.

6. Monitor and adjust: As you begin to follow your fasting regimen, pay attention to how your body reacts and make changes as required. Pay attention to your hunger signals, energy levels, and general well-being, and adjust your strategy appropriately to ensure it is sustainable and beneficial for you.

Overcoming Challenges and Staying Motivated:

While intermittent fasting has various advantages, it may also create difficulties, particularly during the first adjustment phase. Here are some suggestions for overcoming frequent hurdles and keeping motivated throughout your fasting journey:

1. Control Hunger: Stay hydrated, drink calorie-free drinks while fasting, and occupy yourself with activities to help control hunger urges.

2. Address weariness: Get enough rest and emphasize sleep hygiene to battle weariness and enhance peak energy levels.

3. Remain Flexible: Be willing to modify your fasting schedule as needed based on your requirements, preferences, and circumstances.

4. Seek Support: Connect with people who are fasting intermittently to get encouragement, accountability, and support.

5. Celebrate Progress: Recognize and celebrate your accomplishments and milestones along the road, no matter how tiny, to remain encouraged and inspired throughout your fasting journey.

Conclusions:

In this chapter, we looked at how to create a tailored intermittent fasting strategy based on your requirements, preferences, and objectives. You'll set yourself up for success on your path to better health and well-being by taking the time to examine your health objectives, lifestyle considerations, and past experiences, as well as establishing a fasting strategy that is tailored to your specific circumstances. In the next chapters, we'll go over the practical components of intermittent fasting, including ideas, methods, and meal plans to help you negotiate the problems and opportunities that come along the way.

Chapter 3: Intermittent Fasting Methods and Protocols

Overview of Different Intermittent Fasting Approaches

Welcome to Chapter 3 of our examination of intermittent fasting! In this chapter, we'll look at the numerous intermittent fasting techniques and protocols available, providing an overview of each strategy to help you better understand your choices and choose the one that best fits your objectives, preferences, and lifestyle. Whether you're new to fasting or want to change up your existing strategy, this chapter will teach you how to integrate intermittent fasting into your daily routine for better health and well-being.

Understanding Intermittent Fasting Methods:

Intermittent fasting includes a variety of fasting approaches and protocols, each with its distinct approach to alternating between times of fasting and eating. Here's a look at some of the most popular intermittent fasting methods:

1. Time-Restricted Eating (TRE): Time-restricted eating entails restricting your daily eating window to a specified amount of time, usually between 8 and 12 hours, with the remaining hours set aside for fasting. This strategy, known as the 16/8 method, consists of 16 hours of fasting and an 8-hour eating window.

2. Alternative Day Fasting (ADF): Alternate-day fasting is the practice of alternating between days of regular eating and days of fasting, during which you consume extremely few calories or refrain from eating entirely. There are other types of ADF, including modified ADF, which allows you to eat a restricted number of calories on fasting days, and total ADF, which requires you to refrain from all meals on fasting days.

3. 5:2 Diet: The 5:2 diet, commonly known as the Fast Diet, is eating normally five days a week while limiting calorie consumption to 500–600 calories on two non-consecutive days. On fasting days, people usually eat a limited number of low-calorie meals or snacks to produce the needed calorie deficit.

4. Periodic Fasting: Periodic fasting entails fasting for lengthy durations regularly, which might range from once or twice a week to once a month. This strategy may include fasting for 24 hours or longer, with the length of the fast altering according to personal preferences and objectives.

5. Meal Skipping: Meal skipping is a more adaptable method of intermittent fasting in which meals or snacks are skipped as desired or required. This strategy enables people to listen to their hunger signals and change their eating habits appropriately, rather than adhering to a rigorous fasting schedule.

Comparison of Intermittent Fasting Protocols:

Each intermittent fasting strategy has its own set of advantages and disadvantages, so while deciding on the best approach for you, keep your objectives, preferences, and lifestyle in mind. Here's a comparison of some important things to consider when comparing various intermittent fasting protocols:

1. Ease of Implementation: Some intermittent fasting approaches, such as time-restricted eating and meal skipping, may be easier to adopt and maintain in the long run because of their adaptability and less stringent fasting regimens. Others, such as alternate-day fasting and intermittent fasting, may need more

preparation and discipline but have higher potential advantages for metabolic health and weight reduction.

2. Adherence and Compliance: The effectiveness of intermittent fasting is heavily reliant on adherence to and compliance with the fasting regimen. Consider if you can keep to a tight fasting schedule or whether you prefer a more flexible approach with room for occasional lapses.

3. Effectiveness for Weight Reduction: While all intermittent fasting approaches have been demonstrated to promote weight reduction and enhance metabolic health, some may be more successful than others at reaching certain objectives. Choose a fasting program that is appropriate for your weight reduction goals and preferences, whether you want to shed a few pounds quickly or significantly over time.

4. Potential health advantages: In addition to weight reduction, intermittent fasting has been linked to a variety of health advantages, including better insulin sensitivity, decreased inflammation, improved cognitive function, and a longer life. Consider the possible health advantages of each fasting technique before selecting.

5. Long-Term Sustainability: Intermittent fasting relies heavily on sustainability. Choose a fasting regimen that you are certain you can follow for the long term, taking into consideration your lifestyle, preferences, and nutritional habits.

Personalized Intermittent Fasting Approach:

Finally, the best intermittent fasting approach for you is one that fits your objectives, interests, and lifestyle. Experiment with various fasting regimens to determine what works best for you, and don't be hesitant to change your strategy as required depending on your unique requirements and circumstances. By tailoring your intermittent fasting schedule, you'll optimize the advantages of fasting while also enjoying a long-term and pleasurable approach to better health and wellness.

Conclusions:

In this chapter, we've looked at the numerous intermittent fasting techniques and protocols available, providing an overview of each strategy to help you better understand your choices and choose the one that best fits your objectives, preferences, and lifestyle. Whether you choose time-restricted eating, alternate-day fasting, the 5:2 diet, intermittent fasting, or meal skipping, there is a fasting program for you. In the following chapters, we'll go further into the practical elements of intermittent fasting, including suggestions, techniques, and meal plans to help you adopt your preferred fasting approach and reach your health and wellness objectives.

Selecting the Ideal Fasting Schedule for Your Lifestyle

Welcome to Chapter 3 of our adventure into intermittent fasting! In this chapter, we'll go over the complexities of selecting the best fasting plan for your lifestyle. With so many intermittent fasting techniques and protocols available, finding one that fits your daily schedule, preferences, and objectives is critical for long-term success. Whether you're a busy professional, a parent juggling several duties, or someone with a changing schedule, this chapter will give essential insights and practical recommendations to help you establish the optimum fasting plan for you.

Understanding Your Lifestyle and Needs:

Before getting into the intricacies of intermittent fasting regimens, you should consider your lifestyle, interests, and personal requirements. Consider the following variables while selecting a fasting schedule:

1. Work and Daily Routine: Consider your work schedule and daily routine to find the most convenient times to fast and eat. If you have a regular 9-to-5 job, you may choose a fasting schedule that coincides with your working hours and enables you to eat during breaks or after work.

2. Family and Social Commitments: When deciding on a fasting schedule, consider your family and social duties. If you have family meals or social engagements planned regularly, you may need a fasting routine that allows for these activities without creating interruption or difficulty.

3. Exercise and Physical Activity: Think about how your fasting schedule will affect your workout regimen and physical activity levels. Some people like to exercise while fasting, while others find it more pleasant to eat before or after working out. Choose a fasting plan that will help you achieve your fitness objectives and offer enough energy for physical activities.

4. Sleep habits and circadian rhythms: Consider your sleep habits and circadian rhythms while creating a fasting regimen. Aim to synchronize your eating window with your natural circadian cycle and emphasize enough rest and recovery to promote overall health and well-being.

Exploring Intermittent Fasting Protocols:

Now that you've gained a better grasp of your lifestyle and demands, let's look at some common intermittent fasting protocols and how they could fit into your daily routine:

1. Time-Restricted Eating (TRE): Time-restricted eating entails restricting your eating window to a specified time each day, usually 8–12 hours, with the remaining hours set up for fasting. This strategy is ideal for those who have a steady daily routine and eat at regular times.

2. Alternative Day Fasting (ADF): Alternate-day fasting alternates between days of regular eating and days of fasting, during which you consume extremely few calories or do not eat at

all. This strategy may be appropriate for those who have flexible schedules and don't mind periodic full-day fasts.

3. 5:2 Diet: The 5:2 diet consists of eating normally five days a week while limiting calorie consumption to 500–600 calories on two non-consecutive days. This method is suitable for those who want a planned fasting schedule with a few days of low-calorie eating each week.

4. Periodic Fasting: Periodic fasting entails fasting for lengthy durations regularly, which might range from once or twice a week to once a month. This method may appeal to people seeking a more flexible fasting regimen that includes occasional extended fasts.

5. Meal Skipping: Meal skipping is a versatile strategy for intermittent fasting that entails missing meals or snacks as desired or necessary. This method is ideal for those who have unpredictable schedules or who like to eat instinctively based on their hunger signals.

Customizing Your Fasting Schedule:

When determining the best fasting schedule for your lifestyle, you must examine your preferences, objectives, and demands. Here are some suggestions for adapting your fasting schedule to your lifestyle.

1. Experiment and change: Don't be afraid to try out various fasting protocols and change your schedule as required depending on your findings and body input. What works for one person may not work for another, so listen to your body and do what feels right for you.

2. Plan Ahead: Plan your meals and fasting intervals ahead of time to ensure you have the resources and support you need to follow your fasting regimen. Prepare nutritious meals and snacks ahead of time, and share your fasting plans with family and friends to get their support.

3. Stay Flexible: While establishing a fasting plan is necessary, it is equally critical to stay adaptive and responsive to changes in your

habit or condition. Life is unpredictable, so be prepared to change your fasting schedule to meet unforeseen events or problems.

4. Listen to your body: When fasting, pay attention to your hunger signals, energy levels, and general well-being, and make modifications as required to ensure you're getting enough nutrients and feeling your best. You should talk to a doctor or alter your fasting schedule if you're feeling very hungry or exhausted.

Conclusions:

In this chapter, we've looked at how to choose the best fasting schedule for your lifestyle, considering things like work and daily routine, family and social obligations, exercise and physical activity, sleep patterns and circadian rhythms, and personal preferences and requirements. By taking these aspects into account and experimenting with various intermittent fasting protocols, you can create a fasting schedule that fits effortlessly into your daily routine while also supporting your health and well-being objectives. In the following chapters, we'll go further into the practical elements of intermittent fasting, including suggestions, methods, and meal plans to help you adopt your preferred fasting schedule and obtain the best outcomes.

Tips for Transitioning to and Maintaining Intermittent Fasting

Intermittent fasting (IF) has grown in popularity in recent years, both as a weight management method and for its possible health advantages. This nutritional regimen consists of alternating fasting and eating sessions. While the notion of fasting is not novel, the systematic strategy of intermittent fasting has gained popularity owing to its simplicity and potential effectiveness.

Transitioning to Intermittent Fasting:

Transitioning to intermittent fasting may be difficult, particularly for people who are used to eating often during the day. However, with the appropriate attitude and mentality, it is possible to adopt a sustainable lifestyle. Here are some suggestions to help you adapt successfully to intermittent fasting:

1. Start gradually.

Rather than rushing immediately into an intense fasting program, start gradually. Begin by increasing the duration between your last meal of the day and your first meal the following day. This might make it easier for your body to acclimate to prolonged periods of fasting.

2. Choose the appropriate method:

There are various intermittent fasting strategies available, including the 16/8 approach, the 5:2 diet, Eat-Stop-Eat, and the Warrior Diet, among others. Experiment with several ways until you discover one that suits your lifestyle and tastes.

3. Stay hydrated.

Drinking enough water when fasting is vital. This not only helps to prevent hunger pains, but also promotes general health and wellness. Herbal teas and black coffee are also suitable liquids during fasting times, but keep an eye on the additional sugars and calories.

4. Focus on nutrient-dense foods.

When you do eat, focus on nutrient-dense meals that include critical vitamins, minerals, and antioxidants. These include fruits, vegetables, lean proteins, entire grains, and healthy fats. Avoid processed meals, sugary snacks, and high levels of refined carbs.

5. Listen to your body.

Pay heed to your body's hunger and fullness signals. While it is natural to feel hungry during fasting times, excessive pain or lightheadedness may suggest that you should change your fasting plan or eat sooner. Intermittent fasting should not result in acute hunger or deprivation.

6. Be patient.

Results may not be instant, so be patient with yourself as you adjust to intermittent fasting. Your body may need some time to acclimate to the new eating pattern before you notice the desired results. Concentrate on long-term rewards rather than short-term changes.

Maintain intermittent fasting:

Once you've successfully switched to intermittent fasting, the trick is to stick with it consistently. Here are some recommendations to help you maintain your intermittent fasting program for the long term:

1. Establish a routine:

Intermittent fasting relies heavily on consistency. Set particular fasting and eating times that work for your schedule and lifestyle, and adhere to them as much as possible. Creating a schedule might make fasting seem more manageable and sustainable.

2. Plan your meals:

Planning your meals ahead of time will help you avoid impulsive eating and ensure that you consume healthy foods throughout your mealtimes. Batch cooking, meal planning, and having nutritious snacks on hand will help you stick to your fasting plan.

3. Maintain Flexibility:

Consistency is crucial, but so are flexibility and adaptability. Life may be unexpected, and there may be times when adhering to your fasting plan is difficult or impossible. On such occasions, give yourself some flexibility and resume your fasting habit when circumstances allow.

4. Keep track of your progress:

Keep note of your progress and how you feel physically, psychologically, and emotionally while you practice intermittent fasting. This might help you discover any trends or changes that may be required to improve your performance. Consider maintaining a notebook or utilizing an app to document your fasting and eating habits.

5. Focus on Non-Scale Victories:

While weight reduction may be the major reason for considering intermittent fasting, there are several additional possible advantages to consider. Pay attention to increases in energy, mental clarity, mood, and general well-being. Celebrate small successes as proof of your achievement.

6. Seek support:

Joining a network of like-minded people who practice intermittent fasting may provide motivation, accountability, and helpful suggestions and guidance. Having a support network, whether via online forums, social media groups, or local gatherings, might help you feel less alone throughout your fasting journey.

Conclusion:

When done appropriately, intermittent fasting may be a successful and long-term dietary strategy for weight loss and general health. Intermittent fasting may become a seamless part of your lifestyle if you move gradually, use the proper strategy, and adopt healthy behaviors. With patience, perseverance, and a positive outlook, you may gain the long-term advantages of intermittent fasting.

Chapter 4: Navigating Menopause and Beyond with Intermittent Fasting

Understanding Menopause and its Impact on Health

Menopause is an important milestone in a woman's life, indicating the end of her reproductive years. Menopause causes a variety of physiological and psychological changes that might influence health and well-being, in addition to hormone fluctuations. In this chapter, we'll look at the complexities of menopause, its impact on health, and how intermittent fasting may help you navigate this life stage with grace and vigor.

Understanding menopause:

Menopause is a normal biological process in which a woman's ovaries stop producing estrogen and progesterone, resulting in the termination of menstrual cycles. It usually happens around the late 40s and early 50s, although the time varies greatly across people. Twelve months without a menstrual cycle is the diagnostic threshold for menopause.

Perimenopause occurs before menopause and is characterized by fluctuating hormone levels, irregular menstrual cycles, and symptoms such as hot flashes, nocturnal sweats, mood swings, and sleep difficulties. Post menopause refers to the time after menopause when women may continue to suffer symptoms and face long-term health concerns related to hormonal changes.

Effects of Menopause on Health:

Menopause has a wide-ranging impact on women's health, including:

1. Bone Health: Low estrogen levels raise the risk of osteoporosis, a disorder marked by decreased bone density and an increased risk of fractures. Maintaining bone health during and after menopause requires proper calcium intake, weight-bearing activity, and other lifestyle changes.

2. Cardiovascular Health: Estrogen protects cardiovascular health, and its decrease during menopause is related to an increased risk of heart disease and stroke. Managing cardiovascular risk factors such as hypertension, high cholesterol, and obesity is critical after menopause.

3. Metabolic Health: Menopause is often associated with metabolic alterations such as weight gain, fat redistribution, and insulin resistance. These metabolic changes raise the risk of metabolic syndrome, type 2 diabetes, and abdominal obesity.

4. Mental Health: During menopause, hormonal variations may affect mood, cognition, and emotional well-being. Many women endure anxiety, despair, irritability, and cognitive deterioration during and after menopause.

5. Sexual Health: Low estrogen levels may cause vaginal dryness, reduced libido, and pain during intercourse, compromising sexual health and intimacy. Addressing these concerns via communication, lubricants, and hormone replacement therapy (HRT) may enhance overall quality of life.

Intermittent fasting and menopause:

The potential advantages of intermittent fasting in minimizing the effects of menopause on health have received more attention in recent years. While research on the precise benefits of intermittent fasting for menopausal women is lacking, various processes point to its potential usefulness.

1. Weight Management: Intermittent fasting may help with weight reduction by increasing fat loss, maintaining lean muscle

mass, and managing hunger hormones. Given the tendency for weight gain and metabolic alterations during menopause, intermittent fasting may be a useful technique for regulating body weight and improving metabolic health.

2. Insulin Sensitivity: Intermittent fasting has been proven to increase insulin sensitivity, decrease insulin resistance, and improve glycemic management, which is especially important for women experiencing changes in glucose metabolism during menopause.

3. Cardiovascular Health: Intermittent fasting may provide cardioprotective benefits by lowering risk variables such as hypertension, dyslipidemia, inflammation, and oxidative stress. These advantages may help reduce the increased cardiovascular risk associated with menopause.

4. Bone Health: Emerging research shows that intermittent fasting may improve bone health by driving bone turnover, increasing bone mineral density, and lowering the risk of osteoporosis. However, further study is required to better understand the precise processes and long-term ramifications for menopausal women.

5. Hormonal management: Intermittent fasting may affect hormone levels such as insulin, leptin, ghrelin, and growth hormone, all of which play important roles in metabolism, hunger management, and cellular repair. These hormonal changes may reduce menopausal symptoms and promote general well-being.

Practical considerations for menopausal women:

Before commencing intermittent fasting, menopausal women should consider the following practical factors:

1. Consultation with the Healthcare Provider: Women with underlying medical issues, such as diabetes, cardiovascular disease, or eating disorders, should visit their doctor before beginning intermittent fasting. A thorough review may help establish the appropriateness of fasting and guarantee personalized advice.

2. Individualized technique: Intermittent fasting is not a one-size-fits-all technique, and its applicability may vary depending on age, health state, lifestyle, and preferences. Fasting procedures may be tailored to meet individual requirements and objectives, thereby improving adherence and results.

3. Gradual Implementation: Menopausal women who are switching to intermittent fasting should do so gradually and give themselves time to acclimate. Starting with shorter fasting periods and progressively increasing fasting windows may help reduce possible negative effects and improve compliance.

4. Nutritional Adequacy: Intermittent fasting requires a balanced and nutrient-dense diet to satisfy nutritional demands and maintain overall health. Emphasizing entire meals, such as fruits and vegetables, lean proteins, healthy fats, and complex carbs, will help guarantee optimal nutritional intake.

5. Hydration and electrolytes: It is critical to stay hydrated during fasting periods, especially for menopausal women, who are more susceptible to dehydration owing to hormonal changes and hot flashes. Drinking water, herbal teas, and electrolyte-rich drinks can help you stay hydrated and balanced.

Conclusion:

Menopause is an important life transition for women, marked by a variety of physiological changes and health problems. While menopausal symptoms and health concerns are diverse, new data shows that intermittent fasting may help mitigate some of these consequences.

Understanding menopause's influence on health, as well as researching the function of intermittent fasting in supporting metabolic health, weight management, cardiovascular wellness, and hormone control, may help menopausal women traverse this time of life with resilience and energy.

As research into the mechanisms and effects of intermittent fasting in menopausal women continues, ongoing dialogue, collaboration, and personalized approaches between healthcare providers, researchers, and individuals can help to inform decision-making and optimize outcomes during and after menopause.

How Intermittent Fasting Promotes Hormonal Balance

Menopause is a dramatic physiological transformation in a woman's life, marked by the termination of ovarian activity and the fall of reproductive hormones. Hormonal variations throughout perimenopause and the postmenopausal period may cause a variety of symptoms, affecting general health and well-being. This chapter investigates how intermittent fasting (IF) may improve hormonal homeostasis during and after menopause, providing insights into its possible processes and benefits.

Understanding Hormonal Changes During Menopause:

Menopause is described as the permanent end of menstruation, which normally occurs between the ages of 45 and 55, with an average age of 51. It signals the end of a woman's reproductive years and is distinguished by a decrease in estrogen and progesterone production by her ovaries.

Perimenopause occurs before menopause and is characterized by hormonal changes, irregular menstrual cycles, and symptoms such as hot flashes, nocturnal sweats, mood swings, and sleep difficulties. During perimenopause, estrogen levels may vary unexpectedly, resulting in symptoms of estrogen dominance or shortage.

Postmenopause is the time after menopause when estrogen and progesterone levels remain low. Women may continue to suffer symptoms including vaginal dryness, reduced libido, mood swings, and changes in body composition as a result of hormonal imbalance.

Impact of Hormonal Imbalance:

Hormonal imbalances during menopause may have a variety of effects on women's health, including

1. Bone Health: Estrogen promotes bone growth and inhibits bone resorption, which helps to maintain bone density. Postmenopausal estrogen levels fall, increasing the risk of osteoporosis, a disorder marked by decreased bone mineral density and a higher risk of fracture.

2. Cardiovascular Health: Estrogen promotes vasodilation, reduces inflammation, and improves lipid metabolism, all of which benefit the heart. The drop in estrogen levels after menopause has been linked to an increased risk of cardiovascular disease, such as coronary artery disease, stroke, and hypertension.

3. Metabolic Health: Estrogen affects metabolism by controlling energy expenditure, insulin sensitivity, and lipid metabolism. After menopause, decreased estrogen levels are linked to changes in body composition, insulin resistance, and an increased risk of metabolic syndrome and type 2 diabetes.

4. Mental Health: Estrogen regulates neurotransmitter activity and neuroplasticity, which influences mood, cognition, and emotional well-being. Hormonal variations during perimenopause and postmenopause may cause symptoms such as anxiety, sadness, irritability, and cognitive deterioration.

5. Sexual Health: Estrogen regulates vaginal lubrication, tissue flexibility, and libido. Reduced estrogen levels after menopause may cause symptoms such as vaginal dryness, dyspareunia (painful intercourse), and reduced sexual desire, all of which have an impact on sexual health and intimacy.

How Intermittent Fasting Promotes Hormonal Balance:

Intermittent fasting includes cycling between times of eating and fasting, which may have a positive impact on hormonal balance in a variety of ways.

1. Insulin Sensitivity: Studies have indicated that intermittent fasting improves insulin sensitivity and glucose metabolism, resulting in decreased fasting insulin levels and reduced insulin resistance. Intermittent fasting may aid in hormone production management and reduce the risk of hormonal abnormalities linked to insulin dysregulation by fostering more stable blood sugar levels.

2. Growth hormone (GH) production: Intermittent fasting increases the production of growth hormone, a peptide hormone involved in metabolism, tissue repair, and growth. Increased GH levels during fasting enhance fat metabolism, maintain lean muscle mass, and improve overall metabolic health.

3. Leptin and Ghrelin Regulation: Leptin and ghrelin are hormones that control hunger and energy levels. Intermittent fasting may regulate leptin and ghrelin levels, resulting in better appetite control and lower calorie consumption. Intermittent fasting may help avoid overeating by improving leptin and ghrelin signaling.

4. Estrogen Metabolism: Intermittent fasting may change the expression of enzymes involved in estrogen production and metabolism. Studies have shown that intermittent fasting raises the levels of estrogen-detoxifying enzymes. This may help lower the risk of estrogen-related cancers and symptoms of estrogen dominance.

5. Inflammatory Pathways: Chronic inflammation is linked to the development of numerous hormonal imbalances and menopausal symptoms. Intermittent fasting provides anti-inflammatory benefits by lowering pro-inflammatory cytokines and regulating inflammatory pathways. Intermittent fasting, which

reduces inflammation, may help ease symptoms of hormone imbalance and boost general health.

Practical considerations for women:

While intermittent fasting has shown promise in promoting hormonal balance during menopause, women should proceed with care and consider the following practical considerations:

1. Individualized Approach: Intermittent fasting is not for everyone, and the consequences might vary based on age, health status, and lifestyle. Women with pre-existing hormone abnormalities or medical issues should visit a doctor before starting intermittent fasting.

2. Gradual Implementation: Women who are shifting to intermittent fasting should do it gradually and give themselves time to acclimate. Starting with shorter fasting periods and progressively increasing fasting windows may help reduce possible negative effects and improve compliance.

3. Nutritional Adequacy: During intermittent fasting, a balanced and nutrient-dense diet is required to guarantee appropriate nutrient intake. Emphasizing entire meals such as fruits, vegetables, lean proteins, healthy fats, and complex carbs will help with hormone balance and general wellness.

4. Hydration and electrolytes: Staying hydrated during fasting periods is especially important for women suffering from menopausal symptoms like hot flashes and night sweats. Drinking water, herbal teas, and electrolyte-rich drinks can help you stay hydrated and balanced.

5. Symptom Monitoring: Women should keep track of their symptoms and overall health during intermittent fasting and adapt their fasting routine as appropriate. If fasting worsens menopausal symptoms or has a detrimental effect on health, women should stop fasting or consult with a healthcare specialist.

Conclusion:

Hormonal imbalances during menopause may have a significant influence on women's health and well-being, affecting a variety of physiological systems and leading to symptoms such as hot flashes, mood swings, and metabolism abnormalities. Intermittent fasting has the potential to help maintain hormonal balance during menopause by influencing insulin sensitivity, growth hormone production, appetite management, estrogen metabolism, and inflammation.

While intermittent fasting shows promise as a technique for achieving hormonal balance, women should proceed with care and consider their age, health state, and lifestyle. Using a progressive and personalized approach to intermittent fasting and consulting with a healthcare physician may help women endure menopause and beyond with resilience and vigor. As more research sheds light on the processes and consequences of intermittent fasting on hormone balance, continued communication, cooperation, and individualized approaches among healthcare practitioners, researchers, and women may improve results and promote hormonal health throughout menopause and beyond.

Managing Menopausal Symptoms

Menopause is a normal part of a woman's life that signals the end of her reproductive years. While menopause is a natural transition, the hormonal shifts that accompany it may cause several painful symptoms, including hot flashes, night sweats, mood swings, and sleep difficulties. Many women rely on good symptom management to preserve their quality of life throughout and after menopause. In this chapter, we look at how intermittent fasting (IF) might be a useful technique for controlling menopausal symptoms, including possible processes and advantages.

Understanding Menopause Symptoms:

Menopause is defined as the end of menstruation, which usually occurs between the ages of 45 and 55. Women go through perimenopause, a period of hormonal swings and irregular menstruation that precedes menopause. During perimenopause and postmenopause, women may have a variety of symptoms, including:

1. Hot Flashes: One of the most common menopausal symptoms is sudden, acute heat, which is often accompanied by perspiration and flushing of the skin.

2. Night Sweats: Night sweats, like hot flashes, are bouts of profuse sweating while sleeping, which may interrupt sleep patterns and cause exhaustion and daytime sleepiness.

3. Mood Swings: Hormonal fluctuations during menopause may cause mood swings, irritability, anxiety, and sadness, affecting emotional well-being and quality of life.

4. Sleep disturbances: Many women struggle to fall or remain asleep during menopause, which is commonly caused by night sweats, hormone imbalances, and changes in sleep habits.

5. Weight Gain: During and after menopause, changes in metabolism and hormone levels may cause weight gain, especially around the belly, raising the risk of obesity and other health problems.

6. Vaginal Dryness: Lower estrogen levels may cause vaginal dryness, itching, and pain, compromising sexual health and intimacy.

Managing Menopausal Symptoms with Intermittent Fasting:

Intermittent fasting entails cycling between times of eating and fasting, which may have a positive impact on menopausal symptoms via a variety of methods.

1. Regulation of Hormonal Pathways: Intermittent fasting may affect hormone levels such as estrogen, progesterone, and cortisol, all of which play important roles in regulating body temperature, mood, sleep quality, and metabolism. Intermittent fasting, which promotes hormonal balance, may help decrease menopausal symptoms, including hot flashes, mood swings, and sleep difficulties.

2. Improved insulin sensitivity: Research has indicated that intermittent fasting improves insulin sensitivity and glucose metabolism, resulting in more stable blood sugar levels and lower insulin resistance. Intermittent fasting, which stabilizes blood sugar levels, may help minimize changes in energy and mood that are prevalent throughout menopause.

3. Reduction in Inflammation: Chronic inflammation has been linked to the development of menopausal symptoms such as hot flashes, mood swings, and sleep problems. Intermittent fasting has anti-inflammatory benefits, lowering pro-inflammatory cytokine levels and regulating inflammatory pathways, which may help decrease menopausal inflammation symptoms.

4. Weight Management: Intermittent fasting may help you lose weight by boosting fat loss, maintaining lean muscle mass, and controlling hunger hormones like leptin and ghrelin. Intermittent fasting may help lower the likelihood of obesity-related menopausal symptoms while also improving general health.

5. Enhanced Cellular Repair Processes: Intermittent fasting enhances autophagy, a cellular repair mechanism that eliminates damaged cellular components and improves cellular regeneration.

Intermittent fasting may benefit general health and resilience by improving cellular repair mechanisms, thereby easing symptoms of cellular malfunction during menopause.

Practical considerations for women:

While intermittent fasting shows potential as a technique for controlling menopausal symptoms, women should proceed with caution and consider their age, health condition, and lifestyle. Here are some practical concerns for women wanting to use intermittent fasting to address menopausal symptoms:

1. Consultation with the Healthcare Provider: Women who have pre-existing medical illnesses or concerns should speak with their doctor before beginning intermittent fasting. A healthcare practitioner may provide tailored advice and suggestions depending on an individual's health requirements and objectives.

2. Gradual Implementation: Women who are shifting to intermittent fasting should do it gradually and give themselves time to acclimate. Starting with shorter fasting periods and progressively increasing fasting windows may help reduce possible negative effects and improve compliance.

3. Hydration and electrolytes: Staying hydrated during fasting periods is especially important for women suffering from menopausal symptoms like hot flashes and night sweats. Drinking water, herbal teas, and electrolyte-rich drinks can help you stay hydrated and balanced.

4. Nutritional Adequacy: During intermittent fasting, a balanced and nutrient-dense diet is required to guarantee appropriate nutrient intake. Emphasizing entire meals such as fruits, vegetables, lean proteins, healthy fats, and complex carbs will help with hormone balance and general wellness.

5. Symptom Monitoring: Women should keep track of their symptoms and overall health during intermittent fasting and adapt their fasting routine as appropriate. If fasting worsens menopausal symptoms or has a detrimental effect on health, women should stop fasting or consult with a healthcare specialist.

Conclusion:
Menopause is a normal part of a woman's life, marked by hormonal changes that may cause a range of unpleasant symptoms. While there is no one-size-fits-all answer for treating menopausal symptoms, intermittent fasting seems to be a promising technique that may help reduce signs while also improving overall health.

Intermittent fasting may provide several advantages to women going through menopause and beyond by modulating hormonal pathways, boosting insulin sensitivity, lowering inflammation, assisting with weight control, and promoting cellular repair processes. When implementing intermittent fasting into their habits, women should exercise care and consider specific aspects such as age, health condition, and lifestyle.

As research into the mechanisms and effects of intermittent fasting on menopausal symptoms continues, ongoing dialogue, collaboration, and personalized approaches among healthcare providers, researchers, and women can help optimize outcomes and promote health and vitality during and after menopause.

Chapter 5: Maximizing Weight Loss and Body Composition Changes

The Role of Intermittent Fasting in Weight Management

In a society where obesity rates are rising and weight-related health issues are common, effective weight control measures are more necessary than ever. Intermittent fasting (IF) has gained popularity as a viable method for weight reduction and body composition alteration. In this chapter, we look at the function of intermittent fasting in weight management, including its mechanics, advantages, and practical applications for maximizing weight loss and improving body composition.

Understanding weight management and body composition:

Weight management refers to the procedures for acquiring and maintaining a healthy body weight through balanced energy intake and expenditure. While body weight is an essential sign of health, body composition, or the percentage of fat, muscle, bone, and other tissues in the body, is just as important.

Body composition has a substantial impact on metabolic health, physical performance, and general well-being. Excess body fat, especially visceral fat accumulated around organs, has been linked to an increased risk of chronic illnesses, including type 2 diabetes, cardiovascular disease, and certain malignancies. Maintaining a healthy lean muscle mass to body fat ratio, on the other hand, has been linked to better metabolic health, functional ability, and lifespan.

The importance of intermittent fasting in weight management

Intermittent fasting is cycling between times of eating and fasting, which may affect weight control and body composition in a variety of ways.

1. Caloric Restriction: Because of the short eating window, intermittent fasting usually leads to a decrease in total calorie consumption. Intermittent fasting aids weight and fat reduction by producing a calorie deficit, particularly when accompanied by good eating habits and frequent physical exercise.

2. Metabolic Benefits: Studies have indicated that intermittent fasting improves metabolic health by increasing insulin sensitivity, decreasing insulin resistance, and stimulating fat oxidation. Intermittent fasting may improve metabolic processes to help with fat reduction, muscle preservation, and body composition.

3. Hormonal management: Intermittent fasting affects hormone levels such as insulin, ghrelin, leptin, and growth hormone, which are important for appetite management, metabolism, and energy balance. Intermittent fasting may lower hunger, boost fat burning, and aid in weight reduction by altering hormonal pathways.

4. Enhanced fat oxidation: When fasting, the body uses stored fat for energy, which leads to enhanced fat oxidation and ketone generation. Intermittent fasting improves fat reduction and metabolic flexibility by enabling the body to use glucose and ketones for energy.

5. Preservation of Lean Muscle Mass: Intermittent fasting has been demonstrated to retain lean muscle mass while losing weight, which is critical for maintaining metabolic rate, functional ability, and general health. Intermittent fasting may help improve body composition and metabolic health by conserving muscle mass while increasing fat loss.

Practical Applications for Maximum Weight Loss and Body Composition Changes:

While intermittent fasting may be a useful strategy for weight loss and body composition changes, it is critical to approach fasting safely and sustainably. Here are some practical recommendations for boosting weight reduction and enhancing body composition via intermittent fasting:

1. Choosing the Right Fasting Protocol: There are numerous intermittent fasting protocols to select from, such as time-restricted eating (e.g., the 16/8 technique), alternate-day fasting, and the 5:2 diet. Experiment with various fasting plans to see what works best for your lifestyle, interests, and objectives.

2. Prioritize nutrient-dense foods: During meal windows, choose nutrient-dense whole foods, including fruits, vegetables, lean meats, healthy fats, and complex carbs. Avoid processed meals, sugary snacks, and refined carbs since they may undermine weight reduction attempts and harm metabolic health.

3. Keep Hydrated: During fasting times, drink lots of water, herbal tea, and other non-caloric liquids to keep hydrated and avoid hunger. Adequate hydration is necessary for metabolic support, fat reduction, and general health.

4. Monitor Portion Sizes: While intermittent fasting does not necessarily limit the items you may consume, it is important to be conscious of portion sizes and total calorie intake during meal periods. Pay attention to hunger signals, eat gently, and stop when you're full to avoid overeating.

5. Incorporate physical exercise: Combine intermittent fasting with regular physical exercise to achieve maximum weight reduction, improve body composition, and improve overall health. To support metabolic rate, muscular mass, and functional ability, combine aerobic activity with strength training and flexibility activities.

6. Be patient and persistent. Weight reduction and body composition changes take time, so be patient and consistent with your fasting regimen. Instead of pursuing quick results, focus on establishing long-term lifestyle adjustments and celebrating your accomplishments along the way.

7. Listen to Your Body: Pay attention to how your body reacts to intermittent fasting, and alter your fasting routine accordingly. If you suffer from increased hunger, exhaustion, or other negative symptoms, you should reconsider your fasting schedule or consult with a healthcare expert.

Conclusion:

Intermittent fasting is a realistic and sustainable method for weight management and body composition alterations, with the ability to reduce body fat, preserve lean muscle mass, and improve metabolic health. Intermittent fasting may help you lose weight and improve your body composition by causing a calorie deficit, improving metabolic processes, controlling hormone levels, and increasing fat burning.

When following fasting protocols, it's vital to proceed with care and consider individual aspects such as age, health state, and lifestyle. You can improve the efficiency of intermittent fasting for weight loss and body composition by eating nutrient-dense meals, staying hydrated, regulating portion sizes, engaging in physical exercise, and listening to your body.

Intermittent fasting, like any other dietary technique, is not a one-size-fits-all method, and it may not be appropriate for everyone. It's critical to choose a fasting program that suits your interests, lifestyle, and health objectives. Intermittent fasting, with patience, dedication, and a balanced approach, may be an effective technique for obtaining and maintaining a healthy weight and body composition over time.

Strategies for Enhancing Fat Loss while Preserving Lean Muscle Mass

Achieving ideal body composition entails more than simply lowering weight; it also includes reducing body fat while maintaining lean muscular mass. This balance is critical to metabolic health, physical performance, and general well-being. In this chapter, we look at techniques for maximum fat loss while maintaining lean muscle mass, emphasizing the importance of diet, activity, and lifestyle variables in attaining long-term body composition improvements.

Understanding Fat Loss and Lean Muscle Preservation.

Fat loss is the reduction of body fat, which benefits metabolic health, lowers the risk of chronic illnesses, and improves physical attractiveness. However, decreasing weight without regard for lean muscle mass may be detrimental to metabolic rate, functional ability, and general health.

Maintaining lean muscle mass is critical for regulating metabolism, improving physical performance, and avoiding weight gain. Lean muscular mass is a metabolically active tissue that helps with energy expenditure, glucose metabolism, and general metabolic health. Therefore, techniques that promote fat loss while conserving lean muscle mass are crucial for attaining long-term body composition modifications.

Strategies to Enhance Fat Loss:

1. Create a caloric deficit: Fat loss happens when there is a calorie deficit, which means you eat fewer calories than you burn. This may be accomplished by a combination of calorie restriction and increased calorie expenditure via exercise and activity.

2. Prioritize Protein Intake: Protein is essential for maintaining lean muscle mass while losing weight and encouraging satiety. To assist muscle retention and fat reduction, consume high-quality

protein sources such as lean meats, poultry, fish, eggs, dairy products, lentils, and tofu.

3. Focus on Whole Foods: Eat nutrient-dense whole foods, including fruits and vegetables, whole grains, lean meats, and healthy fats. These foods are high in vitamins, minerals, antioxidants, and fiber, which promotes general health and satiety, making it simpler to stick to a calorie-controlled diet.

4. Limit Processed Meals and Sugary Drinks: Reduce your consumption of processed meals, sugary snacks, refined carbs, and sugar-sweetened drinks since these products are often rich in calories, sugar, and harmful fats and may undermine weight reduction attempts.

5. Practice mindful eating. To avoid overeating and increase satiety, pay attention to hunger signals, eat deliberately, and relish your meals. Mindful eating strategies, such as digesting food fully, avoiding distractions, and paying attention to your body's hunger and fullness signals, may help you make better food choices and manage portion sizes.

6. Stay Hydrated: Drink lots of water throughout the day to keep your body hydrated and metabolically healthy. Thirst may often be confused with hunger, so keeping hydrated might help you avoid excessive nibbling and eating.

Strategies for maintaining lean muscle mass:

1. Strength Training: Include resistance training activities like weightlifting, bodyweight exercises, and resistance bands in your workout program to promote muscle development and maintain lean muscle mass. Focus on complex exercises that target several muscular groups, gradually increasing the intensity and volume of your workouts over time.

2. Consume adequate protein. Protein is required for muscle repair, development, and maintenance. Aim to eat enough protein throughout the day, with each meal including a source of high-quality protein. The recommended dietary requirement (RDA) for protein is 0.8 grams per kilogram of body weight per day, although

those who exercise for strength may need more protein to maintain muscle repair and development.

3. Distribute Protein Intake: Instead of eating a huge quantity of protein at once, spread it out throughout the day. This method optimizes muscle protein synthesis while also promoting muscle recovery and repair throughout the day.

4. Prioritize Post-Program Nutrition: Eat a protein-rich snack or meal within an hour of finishing a strength training program to aid in muscle healing and repair. Combining protein and carbs may improve muscle glycogen replenishment and recovery.

5. Get adequate rest and recovery: Give your muscles enough time to rest and heal in between sessions. Aim for 7-9 hours of excellent sleep every night, since it is critical for muscle regeneration, hormone balance, and general recuperation.

6. Managing stress: Chronic stress may hinder muscle development and recovery by increasing cortisol levels, which promotes muscle breakdown. Deep breathing, meditation, yoga, and spending time in nature may all help you decrease stress and preserve your muscles.

7. Keep track of progress: Track your exercises, diet, and progress over time to ensure you're retaining lean muscle mass while shedding body fat. Adjust your training and nutrition techniques as required to reflect your objectives, preferences, and personal reactions to exercise and food.

Conclusion:

Maximizing fat loss while maintaining lean muscle mass is critical for improving long-term body composition and metabolic health. You may improve fat loss while maintaining muscle mass by creating a calorie deficit, prioritizing protein consumption, emphasizing healthy meals, practicing mindful eating, and staying hydrated.

Strength training, proper protein consumption, protein distribution, prioritizing post-workout nutrition, adequate rest and recuperation, stress management, and progress monitoring are all important techniques for maintaining lean muscle mass while losing weight. By combining these strategies with a well-balanced diet, regular exercise, and a healthy lifestyle, you may reach your ideal body composition and sustain long-term success. Remember that lasting improvements need time and consistency, so be patient, remain focused, and enjoy your accomplishments along the way.

Overcoming Plateaus and Challenges in Weight Loss

Starting a weight reduction journey may be motivating and transformative, but it is not without obstacles. Plateaus, setbacks, and barriers are frequent on the route to obtaining your ideal body composition. In this chapter, we'll look at tactics for overcoming weight loss plateaus and hurdles, as well as how to deal with setbacks and remain motivated on your road to a healthier, happier self.

Understanding Plateaus and Challenges in Weight Loss:

Weight-loss plateaus occur when your progress slows and the scale stops moving despite your best efforts. Plateaus may be frustrating and disappointing, but they are a normal part of the weight-loss process. Weight loss plateaus may be caused by many causes, such as:

1. Metabolic Adaptation: As you lose weight, your metabolic rate may reduce, making it more difficult to maintain your current weight-loss pace.

2. Caloric Intake: Over time, your body may adjust to the calorie shortfall caused by dieting, resulting in a reduction in energy expenditure and a plateau in weight loss.

3. Changes in Physical Activity: Your body may become more effective at exercising, using fewer calories to do the same tasks, which may affect your weight loss pace.

4. Fluid Retention: Swings in fluid balance, especially during menstruation or due to changes in salt consumption, may cause weight swings that disguise fat loss progress.

5. Lack of Sleep: Inadequate sleep may affect hormone levels, especially those that govern hunger and fullness, resulting in increased appetite, lower energy expenditure, and probable weight gain.

In addition to plateaus, many hurdles may occur along the weight reduction process, including:

1. Emotional Eating: Overeating or bingeing may be triggered by emotional factors such as stress, boredom, or loneliness, which can undermine your weight loss goals and make it hard to stick to your plan.

2. Social Pressures: Social events, holidays, and parties may all pose obstacles to healthy eating, tempting you to indulge in unhealthy foods or overeat, making it harder to stick to your weight reduction goals.

3. Physical restrictions: Injuries, medical issues, or physical restrictions might impair your capacity to exercise or participate in physical activity, slowing your weight reduction progress and making it more difficult to achieve your objectives.

4. Psychological Factors: Negative self-talk, self-doubt, and body image difficulties may erode your confidence and drive, making it difficult to stick to your weight reduction plan.

Overcoming Plateaus and Challenges in Weight Loss:

While plateaus and problems with weight reduction might be depressing, they are not insurmountable. With the correct mentality, methods, and support, you can overcome barriers and continue to work toward your objectives. Here are some suggestions for overcoming plateaus and problems in weight loss:

1. Reassess Your Goals: Take a step back and review your objectives, motives, and expectations. Are your objectives reasonable and attainable? Are you concentrating on long-term lifestyle improvements instead of fast cures or fad diets? Adjust your objectives to reflect your beliefs, priorities, and long-term vision for health and well-being.

2. Track Your Progress: Over time, monitor your food consumption, activity, and progress to detect patterns, trends, and opportunities for improvement. Use a food journal, fitness tracker, or smartphone app to document your daily habits, exercises, and progress toward your objectives.

3. Shake Up Your Routine: To challenge your body and avoid monotony, try different exercises, activities, or training methods. Include a mix of aerobic, weight training, and flexibility activities in your regimen to keep your workouts interesting and pleasurable.

4. Adjust Your Nutrition: Examine your eating patterns and make changes as required to break through plateaus and conquer weight reduction obstacles. To promote fat reduction and maintain lean muscle mass, consider cutting your calorie consumption, increasing your protein intake, or cycling your carbs.

5. Practice mindful eating. Be mindful of your hunger cues, practice portion control, and savor each bite to keep emotional and binge eating at bay. Mindful eating strategies, such as eating slowly, chewing fully, and concentrating on the sensory experience of eating, may help you make better food choices and improve your relationship with food.

6. Manage stress: Try healthy stress-management techniques like meditation, yoga, deep breathing, or spending time in nature. Stress management approaches may help lower cortisol levels, minimize emotional eating, and increase your resistance to weight loss issues.

7. Get plenty of sleep: Make sleep a priority, aiming for 7-9 hours of quality sleep every night to help with weight reduction, recuperation, and general health. Create a nighttime routine, improve your sleeping environment, and limit screen time before bed to encourage restful sleep and boost your body's capacity to lose weight.

8. Seek Support: Surround yourself with a supportive network of friends, family, or peers who can encourage you, hold you accountable, and guide you through your weight reduction journey. Consider joining a weight reduction group, or an online community, or getting professional help from a certified dietitian, nutritionist, or therapist.

Conclusion:

Plateaus and weight loss issues are frequent on the path to obtaining your ideal body composition. They might be unpleasant and upsetting, but they also provide possibilities for development, learning, and self-discovery. You may overcome hurdles and keep making progress toward your objectives by reassessing your goals, charting your progress, changing up your routine, altering your diet, practicing mindful eating, managing stress, prioritizing sleep, and seeking assistance.

Remember that weight reduction is about more than simply the number on the scale; it's about improving your health, increasing your quality of life, and developing a healthy connection with food and your body. Accept the journey, appreciate your accomplishments, and learn from failures as you navigate the ups and downs of the weight reduction process. Using patience,

With determination and a good attitude, you may overcome weight loss plateaus and hurdles and achieve long-term success on your journey to a healthier, happier self.

Chapter 6: Harnessing Anti-aging Benefits with Intermittent Fasting

Exploring the Anti-aging Effects of Intermittent Fasting

Aging is a natural process marked by a steady reduction in physiological function and an increasing vulnerability to age-related disorders. However, new evidence indicates that some lifestyle modifications, such as intermittent fasting (IF), may have anti-aging benefits and improve lifespan. This chapter delves into the interesting realm of anti-aging research, including the possible advantages of intermittent fasting for delaying the aging process and promoting healthy aging.

Understanding the aging process:

Aging is a complicated biological process impacted by several genetic, environmental, and lifestyle variables. While aging is inevitable, its rate and trajectory can be altered by a variety of treatments, such as nutrition, exercise, stress reduction, and sleep hygiene. hanging is linked to a variety of physiological changes, including:

1. Cellular Senescence: Cellular senescence is the process by which cells lose the capacity to divide and proliferate, resulting in decreased tissue repair and regeneration, cell accumulation is linked to inflammation, tissue dysfunction, and age-related illnesses.

2. Oxidative Stress: An imbalance between reactive oxygen species (ROS) and antioxidant defenses causes cellular damage and malfunction. Chronic oxidative stress has been linked to the aging process and can lead to age-related illnesses such as cardiovascular disease, neurological disorders, and cancer.

3. Inflammation: Chronic low-grade inflammation, also known as inflammation, is a sign of aging and is distinguished by higher levels of pro-inflammatory cytokines and immunological dysregulation. Inflammation causes tissue damage, reduced cellular function, and the progression of age-related illnesses.

4. DNA Damage: Over time, DNA damage accumulates, causing cellular aging and malfunction. DNA damage may occur from a variety of causes, including UV radiation, environmental contaminants, and metabolic byproducts. Failure to repair DNA damage causes genomic instability, which increases the risk of cancer and other age-related disorders.

5. Mitochondrial Dysfunction: Mitochondria are the cell's powerhouse, creating ATP and controlling metabolic processes. Mitochondrial dysfunction, defined as reduced energy generation and increased ROS production, leads to cellular aging and the development of age-related illnesses.

Investigating Intermittent Fasting's Anti-Aging Properties:

Intermittent fasting is an eating pattern in which you alternate between eating and fasting, with fasting protocols ranging from daily time-restricted feeding to alternate-day fasting and periodic fasting. A new study reveals that intermittent fasting may have anti-aging benefits via a variety of pathways, including:

1. Cellular Autophagy: Autophagy is a cellular mechanism that breaks down and recycles damaged or malfunctioning cellular components. Intermittent fasting has been proven to increase autophagy, which eliminates senescent cells, damaged proteins, and organelles, encouraging cellular repair and rejuvenation.

2. Reduction in Oxidative Stress: Intermittent fasting may reduce oxidative stress by boosting the synthesis of antioxidant enzymes while decreasing the generation of ROS. Intermittent fasting may protect against age-related cellular damage and dysfunction by strengthening antioxidant defenses and lowering oxidative damage.

3. Modulation of Inflammatory Pathways: Intermittent fasting has anti-inflammatory properties, lowering pro-inflammatory cytokines and regulating inflammatory path with Intermittent fasting, which dampens persistent low-grade inflammation, may reduce age-related inflammation, and promotes healthy aging.

4. Mitochondrial Function Enhancement: Intermittent fasting has been shown to improve mitochondrial function by boosting mitochondrial biogenesis, improving mitochondrial efficiency, and decreasing mitochondrial oxidative damage. age. Intermittent fasting may improve mitochondrial function, increase cellular energy generation, generation, and protect against age-related decline.

5. Promotion of Hormesis is a biological phenomenon in which exposure to low-level stressors induces adaptive responses that provide resilience and longevity. Intermittent fasting puts cells and tissues under some stress. It does this by activating cellular stress response pathways such as the sirtuin system and the AMP-activated protein kinase (AMPK) pathway. These pathways help cells repair themselves, become more resilient, and live longer lifespans.

Practical considerations for achieving anti-aging benefits with intermittent fasting:

While intermittent fasting appears to be a promising technique for promoting healthy aging and increasing lifespan, it is important to proceed with caution and consider individual aspects such as age, health condition, and lifestyle choices. es. Here are some practical considerations for maximizing the anti-aging advantages of intermittent fasting:

1. Gin cautiously. If you're new to intermittent fasting, start cautiously and gradually increase the length and frequency of fasting sessions over time. Begin with a daily time-restricted food window, such as 12 hours, and progressively increase the fasting window as your body adjusts.

2. Keep Hydrated: While fasting, drink lots of water, herbal tea, and other non-caloric liquids to keep hydrated and maintain cellular function. Adequate hydration is necessary for autophagy, detoxification, and cellular repair processes.

3. Choose nutrient-dense whole foods during meal windows, including fruits, vegetables, lean meats, healthy fats, and complex carbs. ex carbs. Nutrient-dense meals include vital vitamins, minerals, antioxidants, and phytonutrients, which promote cellular health and lifespan.

4. Listen to Your Body: Pay attention to how your body reacts to intermittent fasting and alter your fasting routine accordingly. If you feel exhaustion, dizziness, or other negative consequences, try decreasing your fasting period or breaking it with a small, nutrient-dense meal.

5. Monitor Biomarkers: Track aging biomarkers such as inflammation, oxidative stress, and metabolic health to determine how intermittent fasting affects your health and lifespan. Consult a healthcare physician or functional medicine practitioner.

properly interpret biomarker results and improve your fasting procedure.

6. Combine with other lifestyle interventions: Intermittent fasting may be paired with other lifestyle interventions such as regular exercise, stress management, sleep optimization, and social connection to boost its anti-aging benefits. Adopting a holistic approach to health and well-being will enable you to take advantage of the benefits of intermittent fasting and promote healthy aging from all angles.

Conclusion:

Intermittent fasting has the potential to be a strong tool for promoting good aging and prolonging life by using the body's natural repair and rejuvenation processes. Intermittent fasting may reduce the aging process and protect against age-related disorders by increasing autophagy, lowering oxidative stress, regulating inflammatory pathways, improving mitochondrial function, and boosting hormesis.

When following fasting protocols, it's vital to proceed with care and consider individual aspects such as age, health state, and lifestyle. Starting cautiously, staying hydrated, concentrating on nutritional density, listening to your body, monitoring biomarkers, and combining with other lifestyle changes will allow you to optimize the anti-aging benefits of intermittent fasting and promote healthy aging for years to come.

As research continues to shed light on the processes and consequences of intermittent fasting on aging and longevity, continued communication, cooperation, and individualized approaches among researchers, healthcare professionals, and people may help improve results and promote healthy aging for everyone.

How Fasting Promotes Cellular Repair and Renewal.

In the search for longevity and good aging, the notion of cellular repair and regeneration is critical. Cellular repair and regeneration processes are critical for maintaining optimum cellular function, preventing age-related decline, and increasing lifespan. Intermittent fasting (IF) has emerged as a promising dietary approach that capitalizes on the body's intrinsic ability to repair and replace cells, perhaps providing anti-aging effects. In this chapter, we will look at the fascinating realm of cellular repair and rejuvenation, as well as how intermittent fasting encourages these processes to help with healthy aging.

Understanding cell repair and renewal:

Cellular repair and renewal are vital processes in the body that maintain cellular homeostasis, repair damaged cells, and replace old or defective cells with new, healthy ones. A complex network of molecular regulators, cellular machinery, and signaling channels orchestrates these operations. The key mechanisms involved in cellular repair and regeneration are:

1. Autophagy: Autophagy is a cellular process that degrades and recycles damaged or malfunctioning cellular components such as organelles, proteins, and lipids. Autophagy is essential for maintaining cellular homeostasis, eliminating cellular waste, and fostering cell regeneration.

2. [Stem Cell Activation] Stem cells are undifferentiated cells that can develop into numerous cell types and help in tissue repair and regeneration. Intermittent fasting has been found to stimulate endogenous stem cells, resulting in tissue regeneration and rejuvenation.

3. DNA Repair: DNA repair processes are critical for preserving genomic integrity and avoiding DNA damage buildup, which may lead to cellular aging and malfunction. Intermittent fasting may

improve DNA repair mechanisms and lower the risk of age-related genomic instability.

4. Mitochondrial Biogenesis: Mitochondria are the cell's powerhouse, creating adenosine triphosphate (ATP) and controlling metabolic processes. Intermittent fasting has been shown to improve mitochondrial biogenesis, which boosts the quantity and efficiency of mitochondria inside cells.

5. Cellular senescence is the process by which cells lose their capacity to divide and proliferate, resulting in irreversible cell cycle arrest. Intermittent fasting may help remove senescent cells, reduce inflammation, and promote tissue repair and regeneration.

How Fasting Supports Cellular Repair and Renewal:

Intermittent fasting promotes cellular repair and regeneration via a variety of pathways that are inextricably linked to the metabolic and hormonal changes that occur during fasts. Here's how fasting helps with cellular repair and renewal:

1. Autophagy Stimulation: Fasting causes an increase in autophagy in response to food deficiency and energy limitation. During fasting, cells engage autophagy pathways, which digest and recycle damaged or defective cellular components, facilitating cellular repair and rejuvenation.

2. [Stem Cell Activation] Research has demonstrated that intermittent fasting activates endogenous stem cells, notably in the brain, liver, and skeletal muscle. Stem cell activation stimulates tissue repair and regeneration, which improves cellular function and resilience.

3. Enhanced DNA Repair: Fasting activates DNA repair mechanisms such as base excision repair, nucleotide excision repair, and double-strand break repair. Intermittent fasting reduces DNA damage accumulation by improving DNA repair pathways, thereby protecting genomic integrity and cellular function.

4. Intermittent fasting boosts mitochondrial biogenesis, which increases the quantity and efficiency of mitochondria inside cells. Enhanced mitochondrial biogenesis boosts cellular energy generation, lowers oxidative stress, and promotes overall cell function and lifespan.

5. Reduction of Cellular Senescence: Fasting encourages the removal of senescent cells via processes such as autophagy and immune surveillance. Intermittent fasting decreases inflammation by eliminating senescent cells, enhances tissue repair and regeneration, and delays the aging process.

Practical Applications for Getting Anti-Aging Benefits from Intermittent Fasting:

Incorporating intermittent fasting into your lifestyle may be an effective method for encouraging cellular repair and rejuvenation while also supporting healthy aging. Here are some useful strategies for maximizing the anti-aging effects of intermittent fasting:

1. Start slowly: If you're new to intermittent fasting, gradually increase the length and frequency of your fasting sessions. Begin with a daily time-restricted food window, such as 12–16 hours, and progressively increase the fasting window as your body adjusts.

2. Keep Hydrated: While fasting, drink lots of water, herbal tea, and other non-caloric liquids to keep hydrated and maintain cellular function. Adequate hydration is necessary for autophagy, detoxification, and cellular repair processes.

3. Focus on nutrient density: During meal windows, choose nutrient-dense whole foods, including fruits, vegetables, lean meats, healthy fats, and complex carbs. Nutrient-dense meals include vital vitamins, minerals, antioxidants, and phytonutrients, which promote cellular health and lifespan.

4. Listen to Your Body: Pay attention to how your body reacts to intermittent fasting, and alter your fasting routine accordingly. If you feel exhaustion, dizziness, or other negative consequences,

try decreasing your fasting period or breaking it with a small, nutrient-dense meal.

5. Additional lifestyle interventions: Intermittent fasting may be paired with

Other lifestyle changes, including regular exercise, stress management, sleep optimization, and social interaction, may improve its anti-aging benefits. Adopting a holistic approach to health and well-being will enable you to take advantage of the benefits of intermittent fasting and promote healthy aging from all angles.

Conclusion:

Intermittent fasting is a very effective dietary approach for promoting cellular repair and regeneration while also supporting healthy aging. Intermittent fasting has a significant impact on cellular health and lifespan by increasing autophagy, activating stem cells, improving DNA repair, encouraging mitochondrial biogenesis, and decreasing cellular senescence.

As research continues to uncover the processes and effects of intermittent fasting on cellular repair and regeneration, continued communication, cooperation, and individualized approaches among researchers, healthcare professionals, and people may help maximize results and promote healthy aging for everyone. By integrating intermittent fasting into your lifestyle and taking a holistic approach to health and well-being, you may reap the anti-aging advantages of fasting while also promoting cellular renewal for a longer and healthier life.

Achieving Radiant Skin, Hair, and Nails

Radiant complexions, lush hair, and strong nails are often linked with youth and vigor. While aging is a natural process that has an impact on the health and look of our skin, hair, and nails, a new study reveals that intermittent fasting (IF) may have anti-aging advantages beyond weight management and metabolic health. In this chapter, we'll look at the interesting relationship between intermittent fasting and the health and attractiveness of our skin, hair, and nails, as well as how fasting may encourage radiance and vigor from the inside.

Understanding the relationship between fasting and beauty:

Several variables impact the health and look of our skin, hair, and nails, including genetics, lifestyle, environmental exposures, and nutritional choices. Aging, oxidative stress, inflammation, hormonal shifts, and dietary deficiencies may all influence our skin's health and appearance. Intermittent fasting has emerged as a viable strategy that tackles these underlying issues while also promoting the health and attractiveness of our skin, hair, and nails via numerous processes.

1. Oxidative stress reduction: Intermittent fasting reduces oxidative stress by increasing antioxidant enzyme synthesis while decreasing the formation of reactive oxygen species. Intermittent fasting improves a young look by minimizing oxidative damage to skin cells, hair follicles, and nail beds while also strengthening our integumentary system.

2. Inflammatory Pathway Modulation: Chronic low-grade inflammation, also known as inflammation, plays a role in the aging process, contributing to skin aging, hair loss, and nail fragility. Intermittent fasting provides anti-inflammatory benefits by lowering pro-inflammatory cytokines and regulating inflammatory pathways. Intermittent fasting provides a better, younger-looking appearance by reducing chronic inflammation.

3. Enhanced Cellular Repair and Renewal: Intermittent fasting promotes cellular repair and renewal processes such as autophagy, stem cell activation, and DNA repair. These mechanisms stimulate the regeneration of skin cells, hair follicles, and nail beds, resulting in smoother, firmer skin, thicker, shinier hair, and stronger, more durable nails.

4. Hormonal Balance Regulation: Hormonal imbalances, such as high levels of insulin, cortisol, and androgens, may cause acne, hair loss, and nail irregularities. Intermittent fasting increases insulin sensitivity, lowers cortisol levels, and controls androgen production, all of which promote hormonal balance and enhance the health and look of our integumentary system.

5. Promotes Nutrient Absorption and Utilization: Intermittent fasting improves gut health, increases nutrient uptake, and boosts mitochondrial activity. Intermittent fasting improves nutrition delivery to skin cells, hair follicles, and nail beds, promoting overall health and vigor.

Fasting helps you achieve radiant skin, hair, and nails.

Incorporating intermittent fasting into your routine may be an effective way to achieve glowing skin, luscious hair, and strong nails. Here are some useful recommendations for maximizing the beauty advantages of fasting:

1. Start slowly: If you're new to intermittent fasting, gradually increase the length and frequency of your fasting sessions. Begin with a daily time-restricted food window, such as 12–16 hours, and progressively increase the fasting window as your body adjusts.

2. Keep Hydrated: During fasts, drink lots of water, herbal tea, and other non-caloric liquids to stay hydrated and maintain cellular hydration. Adequate hydration is necessary for preserving skin suppleness, stimulating hair development, and strengthening nails.

3. Focus on nutrient density: During meal windows, choose nutrient-dense whole foods, including fruits, vegetables, lean

meats, healthy fats, and complex carbs. Nutrient-dense meals provide important vitamins, minerals, antioxidants, and phytonutrients, which nourish your skin, hair, and nails from the inside.

4. Include Collagen-Rich Foods: Collagen is a structural protein that helps maintain the health and integrity of our skin, hair, and nails. Include collagen-rich items in your diet, such as bone broth, gelatin, and collagen peptides, to help with collagen production and promote young skin, lustrous hair, and strong nails.

5. Incorporate omega-3 fatty acids: Omega-3 fatty acids are necessary for keeping skin hydrated, decreasing inflammation, and promoting hair development and nail health. Consume omega-3-rich foods like fatty fish, flaxseeds, chia seeds, and walnuts to nourish your skin, hair, and nails from the inside.

6. Optimize micronutrient intake: Make sure you're receiving enough vitamins and minerals that promote skin, hair, and nail health, such as vitamin C, vitamin E, vitamin A, biotin, zinc, and selenium. Consider supplementing with a good-grade multivitamin.

To address nutritional shortfalls, use a multivitamin or tailored supplement.

7. Practice Skincare and Haircare: In addition to dietary changes, establish a skincare and haircare regimen tailored to your unique challenges and objectives. Protect your skin from environmental harm and premature aging by using mild cleansers, moisturizing moisturizers, and broad-spectrum sunscreens. Choose hair care products tailored to your hair type and concerns, and avoid excessive heat styling and chemical treatments that might harm hair follicles.

8. Protect Your Nails: Keep your nails clean and trimmed, and avoid biting or picking at them because this may cause damage and infection. To keep your cuticles nourished and your nails from becoming brittle, use moisturizing hand lotion regularly. To protect

your nails from harm, wear gloves while doing housework or dealing with strong chemicals.

Conclusion:

Intermittent fasting takes a comprehensive approach to enhancing the health and attractiveness of our skin, hair, and nails by addressing underlying causes such as oxidative stress, inflammation, hormone imbalances, and nutritional deficiencies. Intermittent fasting promotes healthy skin, hair, and nails from the inside out by minimizing oxidative damage, moderating inflammatory pathways, encouraging cellular repair and regeneration, controlling hormonal balance, and improving nutrient absorption and utilization.

Intermittent fasting, combined with a nutrient-dense diet, adequate hydration, collagen-rich foods, omega-3 fatty acids, micronutrient supplementation, and a skincare and haircare routine tailored to your needs, can help you achieve your beauty goals while also promoting long-term health and vitality. Accept the power of fasting as a natural, holistic method for uncovering the beauty advantages that exist inside you, and exude confidence and vigor at any age.

Chapter 7: Longevity and Disease Prevention Through Intermittent Fasting

Extending Life and Improving Health with Fasting

In the quest for longevity and maximum health, intermittent fasting (IF) has gained popularity as a dietary approach with several potential advantages. In addition to weight control and metabolic health, intermittent fasting has been linked to improved aging biomarkers, illness prevention, and general well-being. In this chapter, we look at the interesting world of longevity and disease prevention via intermittent fasting, including the processes that underpin its benefits and its potential to lengthen life and enhance health.

Understanding longevity and disease prevention.

Longevity is defined as living a long time while maintaining excellent health and functional independence into old age. While genetics contribute to lifespan, lifestyle choices such as food, exercise, stress management, and sleep hygiene can have a substantial impact. The risk of age-related illnesses such as cardiovascular disease, neurological disorders, cancer, and metabolic syndrome increases with age. Disease prevention techniques seek to reduce these risks and promote healthy aging by treating root causes such as inflammation, oxidative stress, mitochondrial dysfunction, and cellular senescence.

Intermittent fasting and longevity:

Intermittent fasting has been identified as a viable dietary approach for increasing lifespan and reducing age-related disorders. Intermittent fasting has a significant impact on aging, disease risk factors, and general health because it modulates many metabolic and cellular processes. Here are some of the fundamental processes that underpin intermittent fasting's lifespan and disease prevention advantages.

1. Oxidative stress reduction: Intermittent fasting lowers oxidative stress by boosting the synthesis of antioxidant enzymes, including superoxide dismutase (SOD) and catalase, while decreasing the formation of reactive oxygen species (ROS). Intermittent fasting protects against age-related decline by reducing oxidative damage to cells and tissues, promoting longevity.

2. Enhanced Cellular Repair and Renewal: Intermittent fasting promotes cellular repair and renewal processes such as autophagy, stem cell activation, and DNA repair. These mechanisms help to remove damaged cellular components, regenerate healthy cells, and maintain tissue function, all of which contribute to lifespan and good aging.

3. Modulation of Inflammatory Pathways: Chronic low-grade inflammation, also known as inflammation, is a sign of aging and contributes to the development of age-related disorders. Intermittent fasting has anti-inflammatory properties because it lowers levels of pro-inflammatory cytokines, including interleukin-6 (IL-6) and tumor necrosis factor-alpha (TNF-alpha), and modifies inflammatory pathways. Intermittent fasting reduces disease risk and enhances lifespan by lowering chronic inflammation levels.

4. Hormonal Balance Regulation: Hormonal imbalances, such as high insulin, cortisol, and growth hormone levels, are linked to aging and can lead to metabolic dysfunction and age-related

illnesses. Intermittent fasting increases insulin sensitivity, lowers cortisol levels, and regulates growth hormone release, improving hormonal balance and increasing lifespan.

5. Promote Mitochondrial Health: Mitochondrial failure is a major cause of aging and age-related disorders, resulting in decreased energy generation, increased oxidative stress, and poor cellular function. Intermittent fasting promotes mitochondrial biogenesis, increases mitochondrial efficiency, and reduces mitochondrial oxidative damage, thereby improving overall mitochondrial health and lifespan.

Longevity and Disease Prevention with Intermittent Fasting

Incorporating intermittent fasting into your daily routine may be an effective technique for prolonging life and enhancing health. Here are some useful guidelines for maximizing the lifespan and disease prevention:

1. Choose a Fasting Program: Select an intermittent fasting program that suits your interests, lifestyle, and health goals. Common fasting procedures include time-restricted eating, alternate-day fasting, and intermittent fasting. Experiment with various fasting regimens to see what works best for you.

2. Start Slowly: If you're new to intermittent fasting, gradually increase the length and frequency of your fasting sessions. Begin with a daily time-restricted food window, such as 12–16 hours, and progressively increase the fasting window as your body adjusts.

3. Keep Hydrated: While fasting, drink lots of water, herbal tea, and other non-caloric liquids to keep hydrated and maintain cellular function. Adequate hydration is critical for detoxification, cellular repair, and general wellness.

4. Focus on Nutrient Density: During meal windows, choose nutrient-dense whole foods, including fruits, vegetables, lean meats, healthy fats, and complex carbs. Nutrient-dense meals include vital vitamins, minerals, antioxidants, and phytonutrients, which promote cellular health, lifespan, and disease prevention.

5. Include physical exercise: Incorporate regular physical exercise into your daily routine to maximize the advantages of intermittent fasting while also supporting general health and longevity. Choose activities you love, such as walking, cycling, swimming, or yoga, and strive for a mix of aerobic, strength, and flexibility workouts.

6. Manage Stress: Use stress-reduction practices like meditation, deep breathing, yoga, or tai chi to lower tension and increase relaxation. Chronic stress accelerates the aging process and raises the risk of age-related disorders; therefore, reducing stress is critical for longevity and well-being.

7. Get plenty of sleep: Make sleep a priority, aiming for 7-9 hours of quality sleep every night to promote cellular repair, regeneration, and general wellness. Create a pleasant nighttime ritual, improve your sleep environment, and stick to regular sleep-wake cycles to promote restful sleep and longevity.

8. Monitor Health Biomarkers: Track biomarkers of aging, illness risk, and general health to determine how intermittent fasting affects your health. Blood glucose levels, insulin sensitivity, lipid profiles, inflammatory indicators, and oxidative stress markers are among the most common biomarkers to monitor. Consult a healthcare specialist or functional medicine practitioner to learn how to interpret biomarker data and optimize your fasting strategy for longevity and disease prevention.

Conclusion:

Intermittent fasting promotes lifespan and prevents age-related disorders by targeting underlying causes such as oxidative stress, inflammation, hormone imbalances, and mitochondrial dysfunction. Intermittent fasting promotes lifespan by minimizing oxidative damage, boosting cellular repair and regeneration, modifying inflammatory pathways, controlling hormonal balance, and improving mitochondrial health.

Intermittent fasting, along with other healthy behaviors like regular physical exercise, stress management, appropriate sleep, and nutrient-dense eating, may help you lengthen your life, improve your quality of life, and maintain robust health well into old age. Accept the power of fasting as a natural, sustainable way to gain longevity prevent illness, and enjoy the rewards of a longer, healthier, and more meaningful life.

Fasting as a Tool for Preventing Chronic Diseases

Chronic illnesses, including heart disease, diabetes, cancer, and neurodegenerative disorders, are important causes of morbidity and death globally. While genetics affect illness risk, lifestyle variables such as food, exercise, stress management, and sleep patterns all have a substantial impact on susceptibility to chronic diseases. Intermittent fasting (IF) has emerged as a viable dietary approach for avoiding chronic illnesses by influencing numerous metabolic and cellular processes involved in disease development. In this chapter, we look at how intermittent fasting may help avoid chronic illnesses and promote longevity and well-being.

Understanding chronic diseases:

Chronic illnesses are defined as long-term or chronic health disorders that usually grow slowly over time and often have complicated multifactorial causes. The most common chronic illnesses are:

1. Cardiovascular Disease: A variety of disorders affecting the heart and blood vessels, such as coronary artery disease, heart failure, and stroke, are referred to as cardiovascular disease. High blood pressure, high cholesterol, smoking, obesity, diabetes, and physical inactivity all increase the risk of cardiovascular disease.

2. Diabetes: Diabetes is a metabolic disorder characterized by high blood sugar levels caused by insulin resistance or inadequate insulin synthesis. Type 2 diabetes, the most prevalent type of diabetes, is strongly associated with lifestyle factors such as poor food, sedentary activity, and obesity.

3. Cancer: Cancer is a group of illnesses characterized by the uncontrolled development and spread of abnormal cells. Tobacco use, excessive alcohol use, poor nutrition, physical inactivity, exposure to environmental pollutants, and genetic susceptibility all increase the risk of cancer.

4. Neurodegenerative diseases: Neurodegenerative diseases, including Alzheimer's disease, Parkinson's disease, and Huntington's disease, are distinguished by the gradual destruction of nerve cells in the brain and spinal cord. Aging, genetics, environmental variables, and lifestyle factors like poor nutrition and a lack of exercise all increase the risk of neurodegenerative illnesses.

Intermittent Fasting for Disease Prevention:

Intermittent fasting has received attention for its ability to prevent chronic illnesses by addressing underlying risk factors such as inflammation, oxidative stress, insulin resistance, and metabolic dysfunction. Here are some of the primary processes by which intermittent fasting exerts its disease-preventive effects:

1. Improved insulin sensitivity: Insulin resistance is a major cause of chronic illnesses, including type 2 diabetes and heart disease. Intermittent fasting enhances insulin sensitivity by lowering fasting insulin levels, boosting glucose absorption by cells, and encouraging the use of stored fat as energy. Intermittent fasting reduces the risk of type 2 diabetes and insulin resistance by enhancing insulin sensitivity.

2. Reduction in Inflammation: Chronic low-grade inflammation is linked to the development of chronic illnesses, including heart disease, diabetes, cancer, and neurological disorders. Intermittent fasting has anti-inflammatory properties

because it lowers levels of pro-inflammatory cytokines, including interleukin-6 (IL-6) and tumor necrosis factor-alpha (TNF-alpha), and modifies inflammatory pathways. Intermittent fasting reduces the risk of chronic illnesses by lowering chronic inflammation.

3. Increased Autophagy: Autophagy is a cellular mechanism that degrades and recycles damaged or defective cellular components. Intermittent fasting increases autophagy, which eliminates senescent cells, damaged proteins, and organelles while encouraging cellular repair and rejuvenation. Intermittent fasting promotes cellular health and resilience by increasing autophagy, which lowers the risk of age-related illnesses.

4. Reduction in Oxidative Stress: Oxidative stress arises when there is an imbalance between reactive oxygen species (ROS) and antioxidant defenses, which causes cellular damage and malfunction. Intermittent fasting lowers oxidative stress by boosting the synthesis of antioxidant enzymes, including superoxide dismutase (SOD) and catalase, while decreasing the generation of ROS. Intermittent fasting prevents chronic illnesses and increases longevity by reducing oxidative damage.

5. Hormonal Balance Regulation: Hormonal imbalances, such as high levels of insulin, cortisol, and growth hormone, are linked to the development of chronic illnesses including obesity, diabetes, and cancer. Intermittent fasting promotes hormonal balance by lowering insulin levels, decreasing cortisol levels, and controlling growth hormone production. Intermittent fasting reduces the risk of metabolic dysfunction and chronic illness by restoring hormonal balance.

Practical Applications for Disease Prevention with Intermittent Fasting:

Intermittent fasting may be an effective technique for avoiding chronic illnesses while increasing longevity and well-being. Here are some useful guidelines for maximizing the disease-prevention effects of intermittent fasting:

1. Choose a Fasting Program: Select an intermittent fasting program that suits your interests, lifestyle, and health goals. Common fasting procedures include time-restricted eating, alternate-day fasting, and intermittent fasting. Experiment with various fasting regimens to see what works best for you.

2. Start Slowly: If you're new to intermittent fasting, gradually increase the length and frequency of your fasting sessions. Begin with a daily time-restricted food window, such as 12–16 hours, and progressively increase the fasting window as your body adjusts.

3. Keep Hydrated: While fasting, drink lots of water, herbal tea, and other non-caloric liquids to keep hydrated and maintain cellular function. Adequate hydration is critical for detoxification, cellular repair, and general wellness.

4. Focus on nutrient density: During meal windows, choose nutrient-dense whole foods, including fruits, vegetables, lean meats, healthy fats, and complex carbs. Nutrient-dense meals include vital vitamins, minerals, antioxidants, and phytonutrients, which promote cellular health, illness prevention, and general well-being.

5. Include physical exercise: Incorporate regular physical exercise into your daily routine to maximize the advantages of intermittent fasting while also supporting general health and longevity. Choose activities you love, such as walking, cycling, swimming, or yoga, and strive for a mix of aerobic, strength, and flexibility workouts.

6. Manage Stress: Use stress-reduction practices like meditation, deep breathing, yoga, or tai chi to lower tension and increase relaxation. Chronic stress hastens the aging process and raises the risk of chronic illnesses; thus, stress reduction should be prioritized for disease prevention and overall wellness.

7. Get plenty of sleep: Make sleep a priority, aiming for 7-9 hours of quality sleep every night to promote cellular repair, regeneration, and general wellness. Create a pleasant nighttime

ritual, manage your sleep environment, and stick to regular sleep-wake cycles to support restful sleep and illness prevention.

8. Monitor Health Biomarkers: Track disease risk biomarkers such as blood glucose levels, insulin sensitivity, lipid profile, inflammation markers, and oxidative stress indicators to determine how intermittent fasting affects your health. Consult a healthcare physician or functional medicine practitioner to learn how to interpret biomarker data and optimize your fasting strategy for disease prevention and longevity.

Conclusion:

Intermittent fasting is a comprehensive method for avoiding chronic illnesses and improving longevity and well-being that addresses underlying risk factors such as insulin resistance, inflammation, oxidative stress, hormonal imbalances, and metabolic dysfunction. By boosting insulin sensitivity, decreasing inflammation, increasing autophagy, and lowering oxidative stress,

Intermittent fasting promotes hormonal balance, cellular health, illness prevention, and overall lifespan.

Intermittent fasting, combined with other healthy habits like regular physical activity, stress management, adequate sleep, and nutrient-dense nutrition, can help you reduce your risk of chronic diseases, improve your quality of life, and maintain vibrant health well into old age. Accept the power of fasting as a natural, long-term method for avoiding chronic illnesses and boosting longevity, and you will live a longer, healthier, and more fulfilled life.

Reducing Inflammation and Oxidative Stress.

In the search for lifespan and disease prevention, treating inflammation and oxidative stress has emerged as an important technique. Chronic inflammation and oxidative stress are linked to the development of many chronic illnesses, including cardiovascular disease, diabetes, cancer, neurological disorders, and aging. Intermittent fasting (IF) has received attention for its ability to lower inflammation and oxidative stress, hence increasing lifespan and reducing age-related disorders. In this chapter, we look at the processes by which intermittent fasting decreases inflammation and oxidative stress, as well as the consequences for enhancing health and longevity.

Understanding inflammation and oxidative stress:

Inflammation and oxidative stress are closely related processes that play critical roles in the body's response to injury, infection, and environmental disturbances. Chronic or excessive inflammation, as well as oxidative stress, may harm cells, tissues, and organs, leading to the development and progression of chronic illnesses.

1. Inflammation: Inflammation is the immune system's reaction to damaging stimuli such as infections, poisons, or tissue damage. Acute inflammation is a defensive reaction that helps to eliminate the harmful substance and commence tissue healing. Chronic inflammation, defined as persistent immune system activation, may cause tissue damage, organ malfunction, and chronic illnesses.

2. Oxidative Stress: Oxidative stress occurs when the synthesis of reactive oxygen species (ROS) exceeds the body's antioxidant defenses. ROS, including superoxide radicals, hydrogen peroxide, and hydroxyl radicals, are very reactive chemicals that may harm proteins, lipids, DNA, and other biological components. Excess

oxidative stress may lead to cellular malfunction, inflammation, and aging.

Intermittent fasting and inflammation:

Intermittent fasting has been proven to have anti-inflammatory properties because it influences multiple inflammatory pathways and mediators. Here's how intermittent fasting lowers inflammation:

1. Reduction in Pro-inflammatory Cytokines: Intermittent fasting reduces the synthesis and release of pro-inflammatory cytokines such as IL-6, TNF-alpha, and IL-1 beta. These cytokines have important roles in inflammatory and immunological responses.

2. Inhibition of NF-kB Activation: Nuclear factor-kappa B (NF-kB) is a transcription factor that controls gene expression in inflammation, immunological responses, and cell survival. Intermittent fasting reduces NF-kB activity, lowering the expression of pro-inflammatory genes and moderating the inflammatory response.

3. "Stimulation of Autophagy" Autophagy is a cellular process that eliminates damaged or malfunctioning cellular components, including inflammatory mediators. Intermittent fasting increases autophagy, which aids in the removal of inflammasomes, damaged mitochondria, and other causes of inflammation.

4. Boosting T Regulatory Cells: T regulatory cells (Tregs) are a kind of immune cell that suppresses overactive immune responses and maintains immunological tolerance. Intermittent fasting boosts the number and activity of Tregs, improving immunological balance and lowering inflammation.

5. Modulation of Gut Microbiota: The gut microbiota is critical for modulating immune responses and inflammation. Intermittent fasting affects the makeup and function of the gut microbiota, favoring the development of beneficial bacteria while decreasing the prevalence of pro-inflammatory germs.

Intermittent fasting and oxidative stress

Intermittent fasting has been demonstrated to lower oxidative stress by increasing antioxidant defenses, improving mitochondrial function, and decreasing the formation of reactive oxygen species. Here's how intermittent fasting lowers oxidative stress:

1. Antioxidant Enzymes Upregulation: Intermittent fasting stimulates the synthesis of antioxidant enzymes such as superoxide dismutase (SOD), catalase, and glutathione peroxidase. These enzymes remove reactive oxygen species (ROS) and protect cells from oxidative stress.

2. Enhanced Mitochondrial Biogenesis: Mitochondria are the primary source of cellular energy generation and play an important role in oxidative metabolism. Intermittent fasting enhances mitochondrial biogenesis, which boosts the amount and efficiency of mitochondria inside cells. Healthy mitochondria are better equipped to withstand oxidative stress and generate energy effectively.

3. Activation of the Nrf2 Pathway: Nuclear factor erythroid 2-related factor 2 (Nrf2) is a transcription factor that manages the production of genes that help the body fight free radicals and remove waste. Intermittent fasting promotes the Nrf2 pathway, which increases the production of antioxidant and cytoprotective genes.

4. Reduction in Advanced Glycation End Products (AGEs): AGEs are toxic chemicals produced by the non-enzymatic interaction of carbohydrates with proteins and lipids. AGEs promote oxidative stress, inflammation, and tissue damage. Intermittent fasting minimizes the development of AGEs, which lowers oxidative stress and improves cell health.

Practical applications of intermittent fasting to reduce inflammation and oxidative stress:

Intermittent fasting may be an effective technique for lowering inflammation and oxidative stress while enhancing lifespan and well-being. Here are some useful recommendations for maximizing the anti-inflammatory and antioxidant benefits of intermittent fasting:

1. Choose a Fasting Program: Select an intermittent fasting program that suits your interests, lifestyle, and health goals. Common fasting procedures include time-restricted eating, alternate-day fasting, and intermittent fasting. Experiment with various fasting regimens to see what works best for you.

2. Start Slowly: If you're new to intermittent fasting, gradually increase the length and frequency of your fasting sessions. Begin with a daily time-restricted food window, such as 12–16 hours, and progressively increase the fasting window as your body adjusts.

3. Keep Hydrated: While fasting, drink lots of water, herbal tea, and other non-caloric liquids to keep hydrated and maintain cellular function. Adequate hydration is critical for detoxification, cellular repair, and general wellness.

4. Focus on nutrient density: During meal windows, choose nutrient-dense whole foods, including fruits, vegetables, lean meats, healthy fats, and complex carbs. Nutrient-dense meals include vital vitamins, minerals, antioxidants, and phytonutrients, which promote cellular health, decrease inflammation, and counteract oxidative stress.

5. Incorporate antioxidant-rich foods: Eat antioxidant-rich foods, including berries, leafy greens, nuts, seeds, and colorful vegetables, to boost antioxidant defenses and minimize oxidative stress. These foods include vitamins, minerals, and phytates.

Nutrients that scavenge free radicals and shield cells from harm.

6. Reduce processed foods and sugars: Limit your consumption of processed foods, refined sugars, and trans fats, which may contribute to inflammation and oxidative stress. Instead, go for healthy, minimally processed meals that feed your body and promote overall wellness.

7. Include Omega-3 Fatty Acids: Omega-3 fatty acids, found in fatty fish, flaxseeds, chia seeds, and walnuts, are anti-inflammatory and antioxidant. Include omega-3-rich items in your diet to decrease inflammation, improve cardiovascular health, and combat oxidative stress.

8. Incorporate tension management techniques: Meditation, deep breathing, yoga, or tai chi may all help to decrease tension and promote relaxation. Chronic stress causes inflammation and oxidative stress; thus, it's critical to prioritize stress reduction for general health and wellness.

Conclusion:

Intermittent fasting is an effective way to reduce inflammation and oxidative stress, two major causes of chronic illnesses and aging. Intermittent fasting promotes cellular health, lifespan, and disease prevention by modifying inflammatory pathways, strengthening antioxidant defenses, improving mitochondrial health, and lowering the formation of reactive oxygen species.

Intermittent fasting, combined with other healthy habits like regular physical activity, stress management, adequate sleep, and nutrient-dense nutrition, can help you reduce inflammation and oxidative stress, promote longevity, and maintain vibrant health well into old age. Accept the power of fasting as a natural, long-term way to lower inflammation and oxidative stress, and enjoy the rewards of a healthier, happier, more fulfilled life.

Chapter 8: Fine-tuning Your Nutrition for Optimal Results

Designing Balanced Meals to Support Fasting and Well-being

Nutrition is crucial in promoting general health, well-being, and the efficacy of intermittent fasting. Designing balanced meals that offer necessary nutrients, support fasting regimens, and promote maximum health is critical for reaping the advantages of fasting. In this chapter, we'll look at how to fine-tune your diet to promote fasting and overall health, including meal planning, nutrient timing, and food selections.

Understanding balanced nutrition:

Balanced nutrition means eating a range of foods that include vital elements such as carbs, proteins, fats, vitamins, minerals, and phytonutrients in proper quantities. A well-balanced diet improves general health, energy levels, and metabolic function while decreasing the risk of nutritional shortages, chronic illnesses, and inflammation.

1. Carbohydrates: Sugars, starches, and fiber are examples of carbohydrates that are the body's primary energy source. Complex carbs, found in whole grains, fruits, vegetables, and legumes, give long-lasting energy and promote digestive health, but simple carbohydrates, such as refined sugars and processed meals, should be avoided.

2. Proteins are necessary for tissue growth and repair, hormone and enzyme synthesis, and immune system function. Lean meats, poultry, fish, eggs, dairy products, legumes, nuts, and seeds are all excellent sources of protein.

3. Fats are required for energy generation, hormone synthesis, cellular membrane integrity, and nutrient absorption. Healthy fats, such as the monounsaturated and polyunsaturated fats found in olive oil, avocados, nuts, seeds, and fatty fish, should be emphasized above trans fats and excessive saturated fats.

4. Vitamins and Minerals: Vitamins and minerals are micronutrients that are required for a variety of physiological activities, including metabolism, immunological function, and cellular signaling. Consuming a mix of fruits, vegetables, healthy grains, lean meats, and dairy products will help ensure that you obtain enough vitamins and minerals.

5. Phytonutrients: Plant foods include bioactive chemicals with antioxidant, anti-inflammatory, and immune-modulating activities. Consuming a variety of fruits, vegetables, herbs, spices, and teas may deliver a wide range of phytonutrients that promote health and well-being.

Designing Balanced Meals for Fasting and Wellbeing:

Designing balanced meals that support fasting protocols and promote optimum health requires considering nutritional content, portion sizes, meal timing, and food quality. Here are some tips for fine-tuning your diet to promote fasting and overall health:

1. Focus on Whole, Nutrient-Dense Foods: Plan your meals around whole, minimally processed foods that provide vital nutrients and induce satiety. Include a mix of fruits, vegetables, whole grains, lean meats, healthy fats, and legumes in your meals to maintain a well-balanced nutritional intake.

2. Prioritize Protein-Rich Meals: Protein-rich meals aid in muscle mass preservation, metabolic function, and satiety during fasting periods. Include lean protein sources in your meals, such as

chicken, fish, eggs, tofu, lentils, and Greek yogurt, to help with fasting and overall health.

3. Incorporate fiber-rich meals: Fiber-rich meals, including fruits, vegetables, whole grains, legumes, nuts, and seeds, improve digestive health, control blood sugar levels, and increase satiety. Include fiber-rich foods in your meals to help you feel full and avoid overeating during mealtimes.

4. Include Healthy Fats: Healthy fats give long-lasting energy, promote hormone synthesis, and improve nutrient absorption. Avocados, almonds, seeds, olive oil, and fatty fish are all good sources of healthy fats that may help with fasting and overall health.

5. Optimize nutrient timing: Plan your meals and snacks around fasting regimens to improve nutrient absorption. Consume larger meals during eating windows to meet energy requirements, and smaller, nutrient-dense snacks as required to stay satiated during fasting intervals.

6. Keep Hydrated: Drink lots of water, herbal tea, and other non-caloric liquids throughout the day to keep hydrated and help your cells work. Adequate hydration is critical for digestion, vitamin absorption, and general health.

7. Listen to your body: Be aware of hunger and fullness signals, and adjust your meal quantities and timing accordingly. Respect your body's cues and eat consciously to promote fullness, digestion, and general health.

8. Plan Ahead: Take the time to plan and prepare nutritious meals and snacks that are consistent with your fasting routine and health objectives. Stock your cupboard and fridge with nutrient-dense items, and try batch cooking and meal preparation to save time and simplify your meal planning.

9. Be flexible: While it's vital to emphasize nutritious meals and keep a balanced eating pattern,

It's also important to be adaptable and consume a range of meals in moderation. Allow yourself to indulge in occasional snacks and social events without guilt, as long as your diet is balanced and moderate.

10. Seek professional guidance: If you have particular dietary objectives, health concerns, or medical problems, speak with a licensed dietitian or nutritionist for tailored advice and assistance. A trained nutrition specialist can assist you in developing a personalized nutrition plan that complements your fasting program while also promoting optimum health and well-being.

Conclusion:

Designing balanced meals that support fasting protocols while also promoting optimum health is critical for optimizing the advantages of intermittent fasting and maintaining overall wellness. You can fine-tune your nutrition to support fasting and well-being by focusing on whole, nutrient-dense foods, prioritizing protein-rich foods, incorporating fiber-rich foods, including healthy fats, optimizing nutrient timing, staying hydrated, listening to your body, planning, being flexible, and seeking professional advice as needed.

Incorporating these tactics into your daily routine will help you reach your health and wellness objectives, maximize the advantages of intermittent fasting, and eat a balanced, healthy diet that promotes longevity and vitality. Accept the power of balanced nutrition as a foundation for your fasting journey and gain the benefits of enhanced health, energy, and well-being.

Incorporating Whole Foods and Nutrient-Dense Ingredients

Nutrition is the foundation of health, and the quality of our food has a significant impact on our overall well-being. When it comes to intermittent fasting (IF), selecting nutrient-dense whole meals is critical for maintaining metabolic health, enhancing fasting outcomes, and encouraging energy. In this chapter, we will discuss the necessity of including whole meals and nutrient-dense items in your diet, as well as practical ideas for fine-tuning your nutrition to obtain the best outcomes with intermittent fasting.

Understanding Whole Foods and Nutrient Density:

Whole foods are minimally processed foods that preserve their original condition, including vitamins, minerals, fiber, and phytonutrients. In contrast, processed foods are transformed from their natural form by refining, adding preservatives, and removing nutrients, resulting in a product heavy in harmful fats, carbohydrates, and artificial additives.

Nutrient density is the concentration of vital nutrients in a particular diet compared to its calorie content. Nutrient-dense foods provide a high concentration of vital elements per calorie, while low-nutrient meals have little nutritional value compared to their energy content. Prioritizing nutrient-dense foods is critical for achieving dietary requirements, maintaining metabolic function, and promoting overall health and wellness.

Benefits of Whole Foods and Nutrient-Dense Ingredients:

Incorporating whole foods and nutrient-dense products into your diet provides several health and well-being advantages, such as:

1. Optimal Nutrient Intake: Whole foods include a wide variety of vital elements, including vitamins, minerals, antioxidants, and phytonutrients, in their natural form. Consuming a diverse range of

whole meals enables appropriate nutrient intake, which promotes general health, immunological function, and disease prevention.

2. Stable Blood Sugar Levels: Whole foods are often high in fiber, which delays glucose absorption into the system and contributes to stable blood sugar levels. Stable blood sugar levels are critical for avoiding energy dumps, curbing cravings, and increasing satiety during fasting periods.

3. Sustained Energy: Nutrient-dense diets provide consistent energy without creating blood sugar spikes and crashes. Whole foods increase metabolic function, physical performance, and general health by providing a consistent supply of nutrients and energy.

4. Improved Digestive Health: Whole foods include dietary fiber, which promotes regularity, prevents constipation, and feeds good gut flora. A healthy gut microbiota is critical for nutritional absorption, immunological function, and general health.

5. Improved Weight Management: Nutrient-dense meals are naturally lower in calories and richer in satiety-promoting nutrients, making them an excellent option for achieving weight management objectives. By concentrating on whole foods, you may feel content and fed while eating fewer calories, resulting in better body composition and weight reduction.

6. Reduced Inflammation: Many whole foods include anti-inflammatory chemicals, including antioxidants, polyphenols, and omega-3 fatty acids, which help to decrease inflammation and oxidative stress in the body. By including nutrient-dense foods in your diet, you may promote a healthy inflammatory response and lower your risk of chronic illnesses.

Practical Tips for Including Whole Foods and Nutrient-Dense Ingredients:

1. Focus on Plant Foods: Fill your plate with a variety of colorful fruits, veggies, whole grains, legumes, nuts, and seeds. These plant-based meals are high in vitamins, minerals, fiber, and

phytonutrients, and they provide several health advantages for fasting and general wellness.

2. Lean Protein Sources: Incorporate lean protein sources into your meals, such as chicken, fish, eggs, tofu, tempeh, lentils, and low-fat dairy products. Protein-rich diets aid in muscle maintenance, metabolic function, and satiety while fasting.

3. Incorporate healthy fats: Incorporate healthy fats into your diet by eating avocados, nuts, seeds, olive oil, fatty fish, and coconut oil. Healthy fats give long-lasting energy, aid in hormone synthesis, and improve satiety when fasting.

4. Reduce processed foods: Limit your consumption of processed foods, refined sugars, trans fats, and artificial additives, which have little nutritional value and may lead to inflammation, oxidative stress, and metabolic dysfunction.

5. Read labels carefully. When purchasing packaged foods, read the labels carefully and look for goods with few ingredients, no added sugars, and identifiable whole-food components. Look for foods abundant in fiber, protein, vitamins, and minerals yet low in bad fats, sweets, and salt.

6. Shop the perimeter of the grocery shop: Typically, the perimeter of the grocery shop contains fresh vegetables, lean proteins, dairy goods, and whole grains. Concentrate your buying efforts in these areas to highlight nutrient-dense whole foods.

7. Planning and preparing meals: Set aside time to plan and prepare nutritious meals and snacks made with whole, minimally processed products. Batch cooking, meal prep, and meal delivery services may help you simplify your meal planning and have healthier alternatives on hand.

8. Be Mindful of Portions: While nutrient-dense meals provide various health advantages, portion control is still essential for calorie management and weight management objectives. To heed your body's hunger and fullness signals, keep portion sizes in check and practice intuitive eating.

9. Stay Hydrated: Drink lots of water throughout the day to keep your body hydrated and assist cellular function, digestion, and nutrition absorption. Herbal teas, infused water, and coconut water are all hydrated alternatives with added health advantages.

10. Experiment with Flavors and Cooking Techniques: Be creative in the kitchen and try new flavors, spices, herbs, and cooking methods to improve the taste and nutritional value of your meals. Discover new recipes, cuisines, and ingredients to make your meals more fascinating and pleasurable.

Conclusion:

Incorporating whole foods and nutrient-dense items into your diet is critical for maintaining fasting protocols, optimizing nutrient intake, and boosting general health and well-being. Prioritize plant meals, choose lean protein sources, include healthy fats, minimize processed foods, and read

With intermittent fasting, you can optimize your nutrition by carefully reading labels, shopping the perimeter of the grocery store, planning and preparing meals, being cautious of quantities, keeping hydrated, and experimenting with tastes and cooking methods.

Accept the power of whole meals and nutrient-dense components as the foundation of your fasting journey, and enjoy the benefits of increased energy, vitality, and well-being. By fueling your body with nutritious meals, you may improve metabolic health, improve physical performance, and flourish on your fasting journey.

Smart Supplementing to Fill Nutritional Gaps

While a balanced diet rich in whole foods is the foundation of healthy nutrition, it may be difficult to receive all of the necessary elements merely through food. Soil depletion, food processing, dietary limitations, and lifestyle choices may all lead to nutritional shortages. In such circumstances, effective supplementation may help bridge the gap and provide appropriate consumption of essential vitamins, minerals, and other elements. In this chapter, we will look at the necessity of supplementing wisely to address nutritional deficiencies and promote optimum health and well-being, particularly when combined with intermittent fasting.

Understanding nutrition gaps:

Nutritional gaps are deficits or shortages in the consumption of vital nutrients required for good health and well-being. These gaps may occur owing to several circumstances, including:

1. Dietary Restrictions: Restrictive diets, such as vegan or vegetarian diets, may be deficient in nutrients often found in animal-based foods, such as vitamin B12, iron, zinc, and omega-3 fatty acids.

2. Food Processing: Food processing and storage may cause nutrient loss, reducing the nutritional value of foods. Highly processed meals often lack the necessary vitamins, minerals, fiber, and phytonutrients.

3. Soil Depletion: Modern agricultural techniques have depleted the soil, resulting in decreased amounts of key minerals and trace elements in fruits and vegetables. As a result, even foods grown in nutrient-rich soil may have less nutritional value than they did in the past.

4. Lifestyle Factors: Stress, insufficient sleep, sedentary activity, smoking, and alcohol intake may all raise nutritional needs or interfere with nutrient absorption and utilization.

5. Age and Health Conditions: Aging, chronic illnesses, digestive issues, and medication usage may all impair nutrient absorption, metabolism, and utilization, raising the risk of nutritional deficiencies.

To fill nutritional gaps, supplement smartly:

Supplements may help to bridge nutritional gaps and ensure an appropriate intake of important elements. However, it is critical to approach supplementation strategically and target specific nutritional requirements depending on individual criteria such as age, gender, dietary habits, health condition, and lifestyle. Here are some important factors for smart supplementation:

1. Assess unique nutritional needs: Begin by determining your unique nutritional requirements based on age, gender, health condition, eating habits, and lifestyle. Consider pregnancy, breastfeeding, age, chronic illnesses, medication use, and dietary limitations, which may all increase nutritional needs or impede nutrient absorption and utilization.

2. Focus on Key Nutrients: Prioritize supplements that address common nutritional shortages or concerns. Vitamins D, B12, and folate are important nutrients to consider, as are minerals like iron, calcium, magnesium, and zinc, omega-3 fatty acids, and antioxidants like vitamin C, E, and selenium.

3. Select High-Quality Supplements: Choose supplements from recognized companies that follow high-quality standards and are thoroughly tested for purity, potency, and safety. Third-party certifications, such as NSF International, USP Verified, or ConsumerLab, may help assure product quality and effectiveness.

4. Consider Bioavailability: Look for supplements with a high bioavailability, which means they are readily absorbed and used by your body. Choose nutrients that are easily absorbed and accessible, such as methylcobalamin for vitamin B12, chelated minerals, and lipid-based versions of fat-soluble vitamins.

5. Tailor Supplements to Lifestyle: When purchasing supplements, keep your lifestyle and health objectives in mind.

Athletes, for example, may benefit from supplements that promote energy metabolism, muscle recovery, and joint health, while those who are under a lot of stress may benefit from adaptogenic herbs or magnesium supplements to help them relax and cope.

6. Monitor Nutrient Status: Regularly check your nutrient levels using blood tests or other diagnostic instruments to identify any deficiencies or imbalances. Consult a healthcare physician or certified dietician to assess the test results and adjust your supplement regimen as needed.

7. Avoid Mega-Dosing: While supplements may help address nutritional deficiencies, it is critical to avoid taking excessive amounts that may exceed suggested consumption levels or pose health hazards. Stick to the appropriate amounts and avoid mega-dosing, particularly with fat-soluble vitamins and minerals that may build up in the body.

8. Incorporate Whole Foods: Supplements may enhance a healthy diet, but they should not be the major source of nutrients. Consume a balanced diet rich in whole foods, and employ supplements as a targeted intervention to address particular nutritional requirements or deficits.

9. Combine with Intermittent Fasting: If you're on an intermittent fasting strategy, think about how supplements can affect your fasting window. Some supplements may be better absorbed with meals, but others can be taken while fasting without breaking the fast. Experiment with different times and doses to see what works best for you.

10. Seek professional guidance: If you're not sure which supplements to take or how to maximize your supplement regimen, speak with a healthcare physician, licensed dietitian, or nutritionist for tailored advice. A skilled specialist can assist you in determining your unique nutritional requirements, recommending suitable supplements, and tracking your progress over time.

Examples of smart supplements to keep in mind:

1. Vitamin D: especially necessary for those with little sun exposure or darker skin tones, as well as elderly people and those who don't eat enough vitamin D-rich foods.

2. Omega-3 Fatty Acids: It's especially good for those who don't eat enough fatty fish, such as salmon, mackerel, and sardines, or who have a vegan diet.

3. Probiotics: Probiotics are beneficial for gut health and immunological function, particularly for those who have digestive problems, take antibiotics, or have an unbalanced microbiome.

4. Multivitamin-Mineral Complex: Provides a complete combination of vital vitamins and minerals to fill any gaps in the diet, particularly for individuals with restricted diets, weak appetites, or insufficient intake of

Fruits and veggies.

5. Magnesium: Magnesium is essential for muscular function, relaxation, and sleep quality, particularly for those who are stressed, have muscle cramps, or do not consume enough magnesium-rich foods.

6. Iron: Iron is required for oxygen delivery, energy synthesis, and immunological function, especially in those who have iron deficiency anemia or inadequate iron absorption from their diet.

7. B Vitamins: B vitamins are essential for energy metabolism, nervous system function, and red blood cell synthesis, particularly for those who consume a low amount of them or have poor absorption.

8. Antioxidants: Vitamins C, E, and selenium may help counteract oxidative stress and improve immunological function, particularly in those with a high oxidative load or chronic conditions.

Conclusion:
Supplementing wisely may help address nutritional gaps and maintain an appropriate intake of important elements, particularly when combined with intermittent fasting. To support optimal health and well-being, you can optimize your supplement regimen by assessing individual nutrient needs, focusing on key nutrients, selecting high-quality supplements, taking bioavailability into account, tailoring supplements to lifestyle, monitoring nutrient status, avoiding mega-dosing, incorporating whole foods, combining with intermittent fasting, and seeking professional advice.

Remember that supplements should enhance, rather than replace, a well-balanced, whole-foods-based diet. By focusing on nutrient-dense meals and judiciously employing supplements, you can cover nutritional deficiencies, support metabolic health, and flourish on your path to maximum well-being. Accept the power of wise supplementation as an important instrument.

Chapter 9: The Mental and Emotional Benefits of Intermittent Fasting

Enhancing Cognitive Function and Brain Health Through Fasting

Intermittent fasting (IF) is well-known for both its physical and mental health advantages. A new study reveals that intermittent fasting might improve cognitive performance, brain health, and emotional resilience. In this chapter, we look at the mental and emotional advantages of intermittent fasting, including how it impacts brain function, mood control, and mental clarity.

Understanding cognitive function and brain health.

Cognitive function encompasses a variety of mental activities such as memory, attention, learning, problem-solving, and decision-making. Brain health refers to the anatomical and functional integrity of the brain, which includes characteristics like neuroplasticity, synaptic connection, and neurochemical balance. Optimal cognitive function and brain health are critical for sustaining mental clarity, stress resistance, and general quality of life.

1. Neuroplasticity: Neuroplasticity is the brain's capacity to rearrange and adapt in response to external stimuli, learning experiences, and developmental changes. It is essential for memory formation, skill development, and recovery from brain damage or illness.

2. Synaptic connection: Synaptic connection refers to the communication of neurons (nerve cells) via synapses, which are junctions where electrical and chemical impulses are transferred. Synaptic connection is required for brain transmission, data processing, and cognitive function.

3. Neurotransmitters: Neurotransmitters are chemical messengers that send messages between neurons and control a variety of brain activities, including emotion, cognition, and behavior. Imbalances in neurotransmitter levels may cause mood problems, cognitive decline, and other neurological issues.

4. Neuroinflammation: Neuroinflammation in the brain may be caused by a variety of reasons, including infection, injury, chronic stress, or autoimmune illnesses. Chronic neuroinflammation is linked to the development of neurodegenerative illnesses, mood problems, and cognitive impairment.

Mental and emotional advantages of intermittent fasting:

Intermittent fasting has been found to provide several psychological and emotional advantages, including:

1. Enhanced Cognitive Function: Intermittent fasting has been associated with improved cognitive function, such as memory, attention, executive function, and processing speed. Fasting encourages neuroplasticity, improves synaptic connection, and increases the synthesis of brain-derived neurotrophic factor (BDNF), a protein that promotes neuron development and survival.

2. Improved mood regulation: Intermittent fasting may have antidepressant and anxiolytic properties, reducing symptoms of depression, anxiety, and mood disorders. Fasting affects neurotransmitter systems involved in mood regulation, such as serotonin, dopamine, and gamma-aminobutyric acid (GABA), hence increasing emotional resilience and well-being.

3. Reduced neuroinflammation: Intermittent fasting has anti-inflammatory properties in the brain, which protect against oxidative stress and neuronal damage. Fasting, which reduces

inflammation, may help to prevent cognitive decline, neurological illnesses, and mood problems associated with chronic inflammation.

4. Better Brain Health: Intermittent fasting improves brain health by boosting autophagy, a cellular mechanism that eliminates damaged or defective components such as protein aggregates and toxins. Autophagy eliminates cellular trash, promotes neuronal survival, and protects against neurodegeneration, all of which contribute to overall brain health and resilience.

5. Increased stress resistance: Intermittent fasting causes hormetic stress responses in the brain, which activate adaptive pathways that improve stress resistance and neuronal survival. Fasting increases the production of stress-resilience proteins, such as heat shock proteins (HSPs) and sirtuins, which defend against oxidative stress, inflammation, and cell damage.

6. Enhanced Neurogenesis: Intermittent fasting stimulates neurogenesis, or the formation of new neurons, in the hippocampus, a brain area important in learning and memory. Neurogenesis promotes cognitive flexibility, pattern recognition, and spatial navigation, which improves general cognitive performance and brain health.

7. Improved Sleep Quality: Intermittent fasting may enhance sleep quality by regulating circadian rhythms, increasing restorative sleep patterns, and improving cognitive performance. Fasting alters the expression of genes involved in the circadian clock mechanism and sleep-wake cycles, resulting in improved sleep quality and daily alertness.

Practical Tips for Improving Cognitive Function and Brain Health with Intermittent Fasting:

1. Begin Slowly: If you're new to intermittent fasting, start with a moderate approach, such as a 12- to 16-hour fasting window, then gradually increase the fasting length as your body adjusts.

2. Keep Hydrated: When fasting, drink plenty of water and non-caloric liquids to stay hydrated and maintain brain function. Dehydration may affect cognitive performance, emotional stability, and general health.

3. Prioritize nutrient-dense foods: To promote brain health and cognitive performance, eat nutrient-dense whole foods high in vitamins, minerals, antioxidants, and phytonutrients. Eat lots of fruits, veggies, whole grains, lean meats, healthy fats, and legumes.

4. Incorporate omega-3 fatty acids: To promote brain health, neuroplasticity, and cognitive performance, eat omega-3 fatty acid-rich foods such as fatty fish, flaxseeds, chia seeds, and walnuts.

5. Practice Mindfulness: Engage in mindfulness techniques such as meditation, deep breathing, or yoga to decrease stress, improve emotional resilience, and promote cognitive function.

. Mindfulness increases neuroplasticity, enhances focus, and decreases rumination and negative thinking patterns.

6. Get Regular Exercise: Incorporate regular physical activity into your daily routine to improve brain health, cognitive performance, and mood management. Exercise promotes neuroplasticity, boosts BDNF levels, and lowers the risk of cognitive decline and mood disorders.

7. Get Adequate Sleep: Prioritize sleep hygiene by aiming for 7-9 hours of quality sleep every night to improve cognitive performance, memory consolidation, and emotional well-being. Set a consistent sleep schedule, develop a calm nighttime habit, and improve your sleep environment to promote restorative sleep.

8. Seek mental stimulation. To keep your brain active and sharp, engage in intellectually engaging activities such as reading, problem-solving, learning new skills, or socializing. Mental stimulation encourages neuroplasticity, increases cognitive reserve, and protects against cognitive decline.

9. Manage Stress: To decrease stress and boost emotional resilience, use stress-reduction strategies such as deep breathing, progressive muscle relaxation, or journaling. Chronic stress reduces cognitive performance, disturbs neurotransmitter balance, and heightens the risk of mood disorders.

10. Stay Socially Connected: Maintain social ties and cultivate supportive relationships with family, friends, and community members to improve emotional and cognitive wellness. Social involvement lowers the risk of cognitive decline, sadness, and anxiety while increasing the overall quality of life.

Conclusion:

Intermittent fasting has several mental and emotional advantages, such as better cognitive performance, mood modulation, and stress resistance. Fasting can improve cognitive performance, protect against neurodegenerative illnesses, and boost emotional well-being by increasing neuroplasticity, lowering neuroinflammation, supporting autophagy, and increasing brain health.

Incorporating intermittent fasting into your lifestyle, along with other brain-boosting strategies like staying hydrated, prioritizing nutrient-dense foods, practicing mindfulness, getting regular exercise, prioritizing sleep, seeking mental stimulation, managing stress, and staying socially connected, can help you realize fasting's full potential for mental and emotional health.

Accept the mental and emotional advantages of intermittent fasting as a potent tool for improving cognitive performance, brain health, and overall vigor and resilience. Fasting and other brain-boosting habits may help you flourish cognitively, emotionally, and physically on your path to maximum well-being.

Managing Stress, Anxiety, and Emotional Eating Patterns

In today's fast-paced environment, stress, worry, and emotional eating are common difficulties that affect mental and emotional well-being. Intermittent fasting (IF) is a comprehensive method for addressing these difficulties that affect not just eating behaviors but also hormone balance, neurotransmitter activity, and emotional resiliency. In this chapter, we look at the mental and emotional advantages of intermittent fasting, including how it may help you manage stress, anxiety, and emotional eating habits.

Understanding stress, anxiety, and emotional eating.

1. Stress: Stress is the body's natural reaction to perceived dangers or difficulties, resulting in a series of physiological and psychological responses known as the stress response. While acute stress may be adaptive and mobilize resources for survival, chronic stress can hurt health, leading to a variety of physical and mental health issues, such as cardiovascular disease, immunological dysfunction, and mood disorders.

2. Anxiety: Anxiety is a prolonged state of anxiety, apprehension, or fear over upcoming events or circumstances. While occasional anxiety is natural, excessive or persistent anxiety may disrupt everyday functioning, impede cognitive function, and hurt quality of life. Anxiety disorders, including generalized anxiety disorder (GAD), panic disorder, and social anxiety disorder, are distinguished by excessive concern and dread that outweigh the real danger.

3. Emotional eating: Emotional eating is the practice of using food as a coping method for unpleasant feelings such as stress, worry, melancholy, loneliness, or boredom. Rather of satisfying their hunger, emotional eaters may overeat for reasons such as distraction, pleasure, or emotional comfort.

Emotional eating habits may result in overeating, weight gain, and feelings of guilt or shame, creating a vicious cycle of emotional discomfort and maladaptive eating behaviors.

Mental and emotional advantages of intermittent fasting: Intermittent fasting has been demonstrated to provide a variety of mental and emotional advantages that may help manage stress, anxiety, and emotional eating behaviors.

1. Stress hormone regulation: Intermittent fasting regulates the body's stress response by controlling the release of stress hormones, including cortisol and adrenaline. Fasting encourages adaptive stress responses, increases stress resistance, and mitigates the harmful effects of chronic stress on the body and brain.

2. Reduction of Anxiety Symptoms: Intermittent fasting has anxiolytic properties, which serve to relieve anxiety symptoms and increase emotional well-being. Fasting affects neurotransmitter systems involved in anxiety management, including serotonin, gamma-aminobutyric acid (GABA), and endorphins, which promote relaxation and stress alleviation.

3. Enhanced Emotional Resilience: Intermittent fasting improves emotional resilience by encouraging adaptive responses to stress and adversity. Fasting triggers hermetic stress responses in the body, which activate cellular pathways that improve stress resistance, boost antioxidant defenses, and protect against oxidative stress and inflammation.

4. Normalization of Eating Habits: Intermittent fasting may aid in normalizing eating habits and decreasing dependence on emotional eating as a coping strategy. By setting specific meal windows and fasting intervals, IF encourages mindful eating, increases self-awareness of hunger and satiety signals, and lowers impulsive or emotional eating habits.

5. Encouragement of Mindful Eating: Intermittent fasting promotes mindful eating behaviors, including a stronger

connection to food, increased bodily awareness, and intuitive eating. Fasting times help people reflect on hunger, desires, and emotional triggers, enabling them to make more informed decisions regarding their food intake and eating habits.

6. Enhanced Neuroplasticity: Intermittent fasting improves neuroplasticity, or the brain's capacity to rearrange and adapt in response to experiences and environmental stimuli. Fasting enhances the synthesis of brain-derived neurotrophic factor (BDNF), a protein that promotes neuronal development, synaptic connection, and cognitive function, hence increasing stress resistance and encouraging emotional well-being.

Intermittent fasting may help you manage stress, anxiety, and emotional eating patterns. Here are some practical strategies:

1. Establish distinct eating windows: Create distinct eating windows and fasting intervals to help you organize and maintain your eating habits. Consistent meal scheduling regulates hunger and satiety hormones, reducing the risk of impulsive or emotional eating outside of prescribed eating times.

2. Practice mindful eating. Intermittent fasting provides a chance to practice mindful eating by paying attention to hunger, satiety, and emotional signals around food. Take the time to taste each meal, chew gently, and focus on the sensory experience of eating without interruptions.

3. Include stress-reducing activities: To improve relaxation and emotional well-being, include stress-reduction activities in your daily routine, such as meditation, deep breathing, yoga, tai chi, or nature walks. These techniques stimulate the body's relaxation response, lower stress hormones, and promote inner peace and resilience.

4. Keep Hydrated: During fasting times, drink lots of water and herbal tea to keep hydrated and improve cognitive performance, mood control, and stress resistance. Dehydration may worsen stress and anxiety, so stay hydrated throughout the day.

5. Prioritize Nutrient-Dense Foods: Eat nutrient-dense whole foods, including fruits, vegetables, lean meats, whole grains, and healthy fats, to promote brain health, mood regulation, and stress resistance. Nutrient-dense meals provide vital vitamins, minerals, antioxidants, and phytonutrients that promote cognitive performance and emotional well-being.

6. Get Regular Exercise: Incorporate physical exercise into your daily routine to decrease stress, increase mood, and foster emotional resilience. Exercise causes the production of endorphins, neurotransmitters that increase emotions of pleasure and well-being while also helping to reduce symptoms of anxiety and sadness.

7. Seek social support. Reach out to friends, relatives, or support groups to share your experiences, seek encouragement, and get emotional support. Social support reduces the negative impacts of stress, improves coping skills, and promotes emotional well-being.

8. Reduce your exposure to stressful stimuli: Limit your exposure to stressful stimuli like bad news, social media, or toxic settings, which may cause anxiety and emotional discomfort. Establish limits on media usage and emphasize activities that generate relaxation, pleasure, and satisfaction.

9. Practice self-care: Make time for self-care activities.

That feeds your body, mind, and spirit, such as getting enough sleep, spending time outside, engaging in hobbies, and practicing appreciation and self-compassion. Self-care routines refill energy reserves, alleviate stress, and improve emotional health.

10. Seek Professional Help: If stress, anxiety, or emotional eating behaviors continue after self-care attempts, see a therapist, counselor, or mental health professional. Professional help may provide useful insights, coping skills, and resources for successfully managing stress, anxiety, and emotional eating behaviors.

Conclusion:

Intermittent fasting promotes adaptive stress responses, increases emotional resilience, and supports mindful eating practices, providing a comprehensive approach to stress, anxiety, and emotional eating pattern management. Intermittent fasting may help people have a healthy relationship with food, manage stress more effectively, and improve their overall mental and emotional well-being by regulating stress hormones, lowering anxiety symptoms, improving emotional well-being, and normalizing eating habits.

Practical strategies such as establishing clear eating windows, practicing mindful eating, engaging in stress-reduction activities, staying hydrated, prioritizing nutrient-dense foods, getting regular exercise, seeking social support, limiting exposure to stressful stimuli, practicing self-care, and seeking professional help as needed can all help to improve the mental and emotional benefits of intermittent fasting. By incorporating these tactics into your daily routine, you may successfully manage stress, anxiety, and emotional eating behaviors while also cultivating increased resilience, well-being, and energy via intermittent fasting.

Developing Mindfulness and Resilience During Your Fasting Journey

Introduction:

Intermittent fasting (IF) not only promotes physical health, but also gives a unique chance to build mindfulness and resilience, which improve mental and emotional well-being. Individuals who include mindfulness techniques and develop resilience skills may manage their fasting journey with better comfort, awareness, and emotional balance. In this chapter, we look at how intermittent fasting may lead to mindfulness and resilience, allowing people to fully realize the benefits of fasting for their overall well-being.

Understanding mindfulness and resilience:

1. Mindfulness: Mindfulness is the practice of consciously focusing on the present moment with openness, curiosity, and acceptance. It entails paying attention to sensory experiences, ideas, emotions, and body sensations without judgment or attachment. Mindfulness activities, including meditation, deep breathing, and body scanning, promote present-moment awareness, emotional control, and stress resistance.

2. Resilience: Resilience refers to the capacity to adapt, recover, and prosper in the face of adversity, obstacles, or failures. It entails dealing efficiently with stress, controlling emotions, and keeping a sense of purpose and optimism in challenging situations. Resilience is not about avoiding or rejecting stress; rather, it is about building inner resources and coping mechanisms to help you negotiate life's ups and downs with more flexibility and strength.

The mental and emotional benefits of developing mindfulness and resilience throughout your fasting journey:

1. Enhanced self-awareness: Intermittent fasting enables you to develop self-awareness by focusing on hunger signals, eating habits, and food-related emotional triggers. Mindfulness techniques like mindful eating, body scans, and journaling may help

people gain self-awareness and identify patterns of behavior, thoughts, and emotions that affect their connection with food and eating.

2. Improved Emotional Regulation: Mindfulness techniques help with emotional regulation by enhancing awareness of emotional states, decreasing reactivity to stresses, and fostering adaptive coping mechanisms. Individuals who practice present-moment mindfulness and nonjudgmental acceptance of emotions are better able to react to emotional issues with clarity, compassion, and resilience.

3. Reduced Stress and Anxiety: When paired with mindfulness techniques, intermittent fasting may help decrease stress and anxiety by activating the body's relaxation response, regulating stress hormones, and fostering emotional balance. Mindfulness meditation, deep breathing exercises, and relaxation methods all promote relaxation, tranquility, and inner peace, which counteracts the physiological and psychological impacts of stress.

4. Enhanced psychological flexibility: Cultivating mindfulness and resilience improves psychological flexibility, or the capacity to adjust adaptively to shifting situations and internal experiences. Fasting allows you to practice acceptance, nonattachment, and present-moment awareness, which increases psychological flexibility and reduces resistance to discomfort or uncertainty.

5. Enhanced Coping Abilities: Mindfulness practices and resilience-building tactics improve coping abilities, allowing people to face obstacles, disappointments, and cravings with calmer and resourcefulness. Individuals who acquire resilience skills such as cognitive reframing, problem-solving, and seeking social support may successfully handle pressures and failures on their fasting journey.

6. Promoting Gratitude and Well-being: Intermittent fasting and mindfulness techniques build a feeling of appreciation for food, health, and life's rewards. Gratitude techniques, including

gratitude journaling, reflective writing, and gratitude meditation, promote a good attitude, improve life satisfaction, and boost resilience in the face of hardship.

Practical Strategies for Developing Mindfulness and Resilience During Your Fasting Journey:

1. Begin with the aim: Begin your fasting journey with a specific aim or goal, such as improving health, boosting energy, or developing awareness. Setting intentions helps to link your activities with your beliefs and objectives, offering inspiration and guidance for your fasting practice.

2. Create a Routine: Plan a regular fasting schedule and daily routine that includes time for mindfulness techniques like meditation, deep breathing, or mindful activity. Establishing regular routines and rituals encourages stability, predictability, and attentiveness throughout your fasting journey.

3. Practice mindful eating. Intermittent fasting provides a chance to practice mindful eating by paying close attention to hunger signals, meal choices, and eating habits with curiosity and nonjudgmental awareness. Eat gently, relish every mouthful, and focus on the sensory experience of eating without interruptions.

4. Practice Mindfulness Meditation: Set aside time each day to concentrate on your breathing, bodily sensations, or present-moment experiences. Mindfulness meditation promotes present-moment awareness, decreases stress, and boosts emotional resilience, laying the groundwork for mindfulness in everyday life.

5. Cultivate self-compassion: Be kind and sympathetic to yourself as you embark on your fasting adventure, accepting problems, setbacks, and tough times with self-compassion and understanding. Treat yourself with the same respect and attention that you would provide to a friend going through a similar situation.

6. Develop resilience skills. Learn resilience skills like cognitive reframing, problem-solving, and emotion management to help you deal with obstacles and setbacks on your fasting journey. Use

self-soothing methods like deep breathing or progressive muscle relaxation to reframe negative ideas, brainstorm solutions to problems, and regulate emotions.

7. Connect with supportive communities: Seek assistance from like-minded people or groups that share your interest in intermittent fasting and meditation. Connect with others on your fasting journey by joining online forums, and social media groups, or attending local events to share stories, encourage, and get support.

8. Prioritize self-care: Prioritize self-care activities that feed your body, mind, and soul, such as obtaining enough sleep, participating in physical exercise, spending time outside, or pursuing hobbies and interests that offer you pleasure and satisfaction. Self-care refills energy reserves lower stress and increases resilience in the face of adversity.

Conclusion:

Integrating mindfulness and resilience techniques into your fasting journey may improve your mental and emotional health, increase self-awareness, and aid in adaptive coping with stress, anxiety, and emotional eating behaviors. Individuals who practice present-moment mindfulness, emotional regulation, and resilience skills may manage their fasting journey with more ease, balance, and resilience, enabling themselves to access the transformational potential of intermittent fasting for holistic well-being.

Accept the chance to build mindfulness and resilience throughout your fasting journey, remembering that the practice is not about perfection but about growing awareness, acceptance, and progress in the present. By combining mindfulness practices, resilience-building tactics, and self-compassion into your fasting regimen, you may increase your awareness and resilience, allowing you to flourish mentally, emotionally, and spiritually on your path to optimum well-being.

Chapter 10: Overcoming Common Challenges and Pitfalls

Dealing with Hunger, Cravings, and Social Pressures

Intermittent fasting (IF) can be a powerful tool for improving health, promoting weight loss, and enhancing well-being. However, there are benefits and drawbacks to intermittent fasting that are similar to those of any other lifestyle adjustment.

In this chapter, we will explore some of the most common obstacles individuals may encounter on their fasting journey, including hunger, cravings, and social pressures. We'll discuss practical strategies and mindset shifts to help you overcome these challenges and stay on track with your intermittent fasting goals.

Understanding Hunger, Cravings, and Social Pressures:

Hunger: Hunger is the body's physiological response to a lack of food, signaling the need for nourishment and energy. While occasional hunger is a normal part of fasting, persistent or intense hunger pangs can be a barrier to adherence and may lead to overeating during feeding windows.

Cravings: Cravings are intense desires or urges to consume specific foods, often driven by psychological, emotional, or environmental factors rather than genuine hunger. Cravings can be triggered by stress, boredom, social cues, or conditioned associations with certain foods, making them challenging to resist, especially during fasting periods.

Social Pressures: Social pressures are external influences from friends, family, coworkers, or other social situations that may conflict with your fasting goals or dietary preferences. Social pressures can manifest in the form of peer pressure to eat, cultural expectations around food, or social events centered on food consumption, posing challenges to fasting adherence.

Overcoming Hunger, Cravings, and Social Pressures:

Understand the Difference Between Hunger and Cravings: Learn to distinguish between physical hunger and emotional cravings. Physical hunger typically arises gradually and is accompanied by stomach growling, weakness, or lightheadedness, while cravings are often sudden, intense, and specific to certain foods.

Stay Hydrated: Drink plenty of water, herbal tea, or black coffee during fasting periods to stay hydrated and help suppress appetite. Dehydration can exacerbate feelings of hunger, so it's essential to prioritize fluid intake throughout the day.

Choose Filling Foods: Opt for nutrient-dense, high-fiber foods that promote satiety and keep you feeling full longer. Include plenty of fruits, vegetables, whole grains, lean proteins, and healthy fats in your meals to help curb hunger and prevent overeating.

Experiment with various fasting methods: Explore different fasting protocols, such as time-restricted feeding, alternate-day fasting, or extended fasting, to find the approach that works best for your lifestyle and preferences. Experimenting with different fasting schedules can help you identify the most sustainable and effective strategy for managing hunger and cravings.

Practice mindful eating. Use intermittent fasting as an opportunity to practice mindful eating, paying attention to hunger cues, food choices, and eating behaviors with awareness and nonjudgmental acceptance. Eat slowly, savor each bite, and tune into the sensory experience of eating without distractions.

Plan for social events: Anticipate social pressures, and plan for social events or gatherings where food may be a focal point. In advance, communicate your fasting goals and dietary preferences to friends and family members, and consider bringing a dish or snack that aligns with your fasting plan.

Set Boundaries: Assertively communicate your boundaries and priorities when faced with social pressures to eat outside of your fasting window. Politely decline food offerings or invitations to eat if they conflict with your fasting goals, and offer alternative ways to connect or socialize that don't revolve around food.

Seek Support: Surround yourself with a supportive community of like-minded individuals who share your fasting goals and can offer encouragement, advice, and accountability. Join online forums, social media groups, or local meetups to connect with others on similar fasting journeys.

Practice Self-Compassion: Be gentle and compassionate with yourself as you navigate challenges and setbacks on your fasting journey. Acknowledge that occasional hunger, cravings, or deviations from your fasting plan are normal and part of the learning process. Treat yourself with love and empathy rather than judgment. Focus on non-food activities: During fasting periods, turn your attention away from food-related activities or triggers and engage in non-food-related hobbies, interests, or social activities. Stay busy with activities such as reading, exercise, meditation, hobbies, or spending time with loved ones to distract yourself from hunger or cravings.

Conclusion:

Overcoming common challenges and pitfalls such as hunger, cravings, and social pressures is an integral part of the intermittent fasting journey. By understanding the underlying causes of these challenges and implementing practical strategies to address them, you can enhance your fasting adherence, promote long-term success, and reap the many health benefits of intermittent fasting.

Remember that intermittent fasting is a flexible and adaptable approach to eating that can be customized to suit your individual needs, preferences, and lifestyle. Stay patient, stay persistent, and stay focused on your goals as you navigate the ups and downs of your fasting journey. With mindfulness, resilience, and a supportive mindset, you can overcome challenges, cultivate a positive relationship with food, and achieve sustainable success on your intermittent fasting journey.

Troubleshooting common issues during intermittent fasting

Intermittent fasting (IF) has gained popularity as a lifestyle approach for weight management, metabolic health, and overall well-being. While IF offers numerous benefits, individuals may encounter common challenges and pitfalls along their fasting journey. In this chapter, we will delve into troubleshooting strategies for addressing common issues such as plateaus, fatigue, digestive issues, and mood fluctuations during intermittent fasting. By understanding these challenges and implementing practical solutions, individuals can optimize their fasting experience and achieve their health and wellness goals.

Identifying common issues during intermittent fasting:

Plateaus: Plateaus occur when weight loss or other health improvements stall despite consistent adherence to an intermittent fasting regimen. Plateaus can be frustrating and demotivating, leading individuals to question the effectiveness of their fasting approach.

Fatigue: Some people may experience fatigue or low energy levels during fasting periods, particularly when transitioning to a new fasting schedule or prolonged fasting durations. Fatigue can impact daily functioning and hinder productivity and enjoyment of activities.

When starting intermittent fasting or making dietary changes, digestive issues such as bloating, gas, constipation, or diarrhea may arise. These issues can disrupt digestion, cause discomfort, and impact overall well-being.

Mood Fluctuations: Changes in mood, such as irritability, anxiety, or mood swings, may occur during intermittent fasting, particularly during fasting periods or when experiencing hunger or cravings. Mood fluctuations can affect interpersonal relationships, work performance, and the overall quality of life.

Troubleshooting common issues during intermittent fasting:

Plateaus:

Evaluate Caloric Intake: Assess your caloric intake during feeding windows to ensure you are consuming an appropriate number of calories for your energy needs. It's possible that consuming too many calories, even within a restricted eating window, could contribute to a weight loss plateau.

Review Macronutrient Balance: Pay attention to the macronutrient composition of your meals, focusing on adequate protein intake to support muscle maintenance and metabolic rate. Adjusting your macronutrient balance, such as increasing protein and reducing carbohydrates, may help you break through a plateau.

Incorporate Periodic Calorie Cycling: Consider incorporating periodic calorie cycling into your fasting regimen, alternating between higher and lower calorie days, to prevent metabolic adaptation and stimulate fat loss. This approach can help you overcome plateaus and promote continued progress toward your goals.

Modify the Fasting Protocol: Experiment with different fasting protocols, such as adjusting fasting duration, frequency, or timing of meals, to break through a weight loss plateau. Changing your fasting routine can keep your metabolism guessing and prevent adaptation to a specific fasting pattern.

Fatigue:

Ensure Sufficient Hydration: Stay hydrated throughout the day by drinking water, herbal tea, or electrolyte-rich beverages to support hydration and energy levels during fasting periods. Dehydration can exacerbate fatigue, so it's essential to prioritize fluid intake.

Prioritize Electrolyte Balance: Pay attention to electrolyte balance by consuming foods rich in sodium, potassium, magnesium, and calcium to support hydration, muscle function, and energy production. Consider supplementing with electrolytes if needed, especially during prolonged fasting or intense exercise.

Optimize Sleep Quality: Prioritize sleep hygiene and aim for 7-9 hours of quality sleep per night to support energy levels, cognitive function, and mood regulation. Create a relaxing bedtime routine, optimize your sleep environment, and establish a consistent restorative sleep schedule.

Managing stress levels: Practice stress management techniques such as mindfulness meditation, deep breathing exercises, or yoga to reduce stress levels and promote relaxation. Chronic stress can contribute to fatigue and energy depletion, so it's important to prioritize stress reduction.

Digestive Issues:

Identify trigger foods: Pay attention to your diet and identify trigger foods that may exacerbate digestive issues, such as gluten, dairy, or high-FODMAP foods. Eliminating or reducing these trigger foods from your diet may alleviate digestive discomfort and improve symptoms.

Gradually Introduce Fiber: To support digestive health and regularity, gradually increase your fiber intake by incorporating fiber-rich foods such as fruits, vegetables, whole grains, and legumes into your meals. Be mindful of your body's response and adjust fiber intake as needed to avoid discomfort.

Stay Hydrated: Drink plenty of water throughout the day to support hydration and facilitate proper digestion. Adequate hydration helps soften stool, promote bowel movements, and prevent constipation or digestive issues.

Consider Digestive Enzymes or Probiotics: Supplementing with digestive enzymes or probiotics may help support digestive health, improve nutrient absorption, and alleviate symptoms of bloating, gas, or indigestion.

Mood Fluctuations

Practice stress-reduction techniques: Engage in stress-reduction techniques such as mindfulness meditation, deep breathing exercises, or progressive muscle relaxation to manage stress levels and promote emotional well-being. Stress reduction techniques can help alleviate mood fluctuations and promote a sense of calm and balance.

Stay Connected: Maintain social connections and seek support from friends, family, or support groups to cope with mood fluctuations and emotional challenges. Sharing your experiences, expressing emotions, and receiving support from others can help improve mood and reduce feelings of isolation or loneliness.

Prioritize self-care: Prioritize self-care activities that nourish your body, mind, and soul, such as exercise, hobbies, relaxation, or creative expression. Taking time for self-care can help reduce stress, improve mood, and promote overall well-being during intermittent fasting.

Address Underlying Factors: If mood fluctuations persist or worsen, consider consulting with a healthcare professional to address any underlying factors contributing to mood disturbances, such as hormonal imbalances, nutritional deficiencies, or mental health conditions. A healthcare professional can provide personalized recommendations and support to help manage mood fluctuations effectively.

Conclusion:

Navigating common challenges and pitfalls during intermittent fasting requires patience, persistence, and a proactive approach to problem-solving. By identifying potential issues such as plateaus, fatigue, digestive issues, and mood fluctuations, and implementing practical strategies to address them, individuals can optimize their fasting experience and achieve their health and wellness goals.

Remember that intermittent fasting is a flexible and adaptable approach to eating that can be customized to suit individual needs, preferences, and lifestyles. Stay open-minded, stay curious, and stay committed to your fasting journey, knowing that overcoming challenges is an integral part of the process. With perseverance, resilience, and a positive mindset, you can troubleshoot common issues and unlock the transformative potential of intermittent fasting for improved health, vitality, and well-being.

Staying Motivated and Consistent for Long-term Success

Introduction:

Embarking on an intermittent fasting journey can bring about numerous health benefits, but it also presents challenges that may test your commitment and resolve. Maintaining motivation and consistency over the long term is essential for achieving sustained success with intermittent fasting. In this chapter, we'll explore practical strategies and mindset shifts to help you stay motivated, overcome obstacles, and maintain consistency on your fasting journey.

Understanding motivation and consistency:

Motivation: Motivation is the driving force behind our actions and behaviors. It encompasses the desire, energy, and enthusiasm to pursue goals, overcome challenges, and achieve desired outcomes. Motivation can be influenced by internal factors such as values, beliefs, and goals, as well as external factors such as social support, accountability, and rewards.

Consistency: Consistency refers to the ability to maintain regularity, adherence, and persistence in behaviors or habits over time. Consistency is key to achieving long-term success with intermittent fasting, as it allows for the accumulation of positive habits, progress, and results over time. Consistent adherence to fasting protocols and lifestyle habits is essential for maximizing benefits and sustaining positive changes.

Maintaining motivation and consistency for long-term success:

Clarify Your Why: Start by clarifying your reasons for pursuing intermittent fasting and your desired outcomes. Reflect on the health benefits, personal goals, or values that motivate you to embark on this journey. Having a clear sense of purpose and direction can fuel your motivation and provide a sense of meaning and commitment to your fasting practice.

Set SMART Goals: Establish specific, measurable, achievable, relevant, and time-bound (SMART) goals related to your intermittent fasting journey. Break down larger goals into smaller, manageable milestones that you can track and celebrate along the way. Setting SMART goals provides clarity, focus, and accountability, increasing your motivation and commitment to your fasting regimen.

Create a supportive environment: Surround yourself with a supportive environment that fosters your fasting goals and encourages positive behaviors. Seek support from friends, family members, or online communities that share similar health and wellness goals. Surround yourself with people who uplift, encourage, and inspire you to stay motivated and consistent on your fasting journey.

Find Your Why Beyond Weight Loss: While weight loss may be a common motivation for starting intermittent fasting, it's essential to identify additional reasons for pursuing this lifestyle. Consider the broader health benefits, such as improved metabolic health, increased energy levels, enhanced mental clarity, and longevity. Finding intrinsic motivations beyond weight loss can sustain your commitment to intermittent fasting even when progress stalls or challenges arise.

Track Your Progress: Keep track of your progress, achievements, and milestones throughout your intermittent fasting journey. Use tools such as a fasting journal, mobile apps, or wearable devices to monitor fasting schedules, eating patterns, and health metrics. Tracking your progress provides tangible evidence of your efforts and accomplishments, boosting your confidence, motivation, and sense of achievement.

Celebrate Small Wins: Celebrate your successes, no matter how small, and acknowledge your progress along the way. Whether it's reaching a fasting milestone, sticking to your eating window, or resisting temptation during a challenging moment, take time to acknowledge and celebrate your achievements. Celebrating small wins reinforces positive behaviors, boosts self-confidence, and reinforces your commitment to intermittent fasting.

Practice Self-Compassion: Be kind and compassionate with yourself as you navigate challenges, setbacks, and moments of difficulty on your fasting journey. Embrace imperfection and view setbacks as opportunities for growth and learning rather than reasons for self-criticism or judgment. Practice self-compassion by offering yourself kindness, understanding, and support during challenging times.

Visualize Success: Using visualization techniques, imagine yourself achieving your desired outcomes and living your best life as a result of intermittent fasting. Create a mental image of yourself feeling healthy, vibrant, and confident, and visualize the positive impact of intermittent fasting on your health, well-being, and quality of life. Visualization can help reinforce your motivation, increase your confidence, and keep you focused on your goals.

Stay Flexible and Adapt: Remain flexible and adaptable in your approach to intermittent fasting, recognizing that progress may not always follow a linear path. Be willing to adjust your fasting schedule, dietary choices, or lifestyle habits as needed to accommodate changes in circumstances, preferences, or goals. Staying flexible allows you to navigate obstacles, overcome challenges, and maintain consistency in the face of adversity.

Practice Gratitude: Cultivate an attitude of gratitude for the opportunity to pursue intermittent fasting and improve your health and well-being. Take time each day to express gratitude for the progress you've made, the support you've received, and the blessings in your life. Practicing gratitude fosters a positive mindset, enhances resilience, and reinforces your motivation to continue your fasting journey with enthusiasm and appreciation.

Conclusion:

Staying motivated and consistent for long-term success with intermittent fasting requires commitment, resilience, and a positive mindset.

. By clarifying your reasons for pursuing intermittent fasting, setting SMART goals, creating a supportive environment, finding intrinsic motivations, tracking your progress, celebrating small wins, practicing self-compassion, visualizing success, staying flexible and adaptable, and practicing gratitude, you can sustain your motivation and commitment over time.

Remember that intermittent fasting is a journey, not a destination, and progress may unfold gradually over time. Embrace the process, stay patient, and stay focused on your goals, knowing that every step forward brings you closer to the health, vitality, and well-being you desire. With perseverance, determination, and a supportive mindset, you can overcome challenges, achieve your goals, and experience the transformative benefits of intermittent fasting for a healthier, happier life.

Chapter 11: Sustainable Living and Intermittent Fasting

Aligning Fasting Practices with Environmental Sustainability

Intermittent fasting (IF) has various health advantages, but its influence goes beyond personal well-being to larger environmental issues. As people aspire to live more sustainable lives, it is critical to investigate how fasting habits might be aligned with environmental values. In this chapter, we will look at the relationship between intermittent fasting and sustainable living, specifically how to reduce environmental impact while enjoying the health benefits of fasting.

Understanding Sustainability and Intermittent Fasting:

1. Sustainable living: Sustainable living entails making decisions and engaging in actions that reduce environmental damage, preserve natural resources, and promote long-term ecological balance. Sustainable living involves many areas of everyday life, such as consumption, energy usage, transportation, waste management, and food production.

2. Intermittent Fasting: Intermittent fasting is a kind of eating pattern in which fasting and eating periods alternate. It provides health advantages such as weight reduction, better metabolic health, greater cellular repair, and an increased lifespan. While intermittent fasting is mainly concerned with human health

outcomes, its implications for environmental sustainability are being acknowledged and investigated.

Aligning Fasting Practices and Environmental Sustainability:

1. Reduced Food Waste:

Plan Your Meals Mindfully: Plan your meals carefully to save food waste and utilize perishable foods before they deteriorate. To reduce food waste, make creative use of leftovers, use flexible items, and emphasize meal planning.

Optimize Portion Sizes: To avoid overconsumption and waste, use portion control. To reduce leftovers, serve in smaller quantities and use smaller dishes and bowls.

Compost Food Scraps: Use food scraps like fruit and vegetable peels, coffee grinds, and eggshells to remove organic waste from landfills while also producing nutrient-rich soil for gardening. Composting decreases methane emissions while improving soil health and fertility.

2. Selecting sustainable foods:

Emphasize Plant-Based Foods: To lessen the environmental impact of your meals, prioritize plant-based foods such as fruits, vegetables, legumes, whole grains, nuts, and seeds. Plant-based diets consume fewer natural resources and generate fewer greenhouse gas emissions than animal-based diets.

Promote Local and Sustainable Agriculture: Help local farmers markets, community-supported agriculture (CSA) programs, and sustainable food producers cut food miles, boost local economies, and promote environmentally friendly agricultural techniques.

Reduce Packaging Waste: Where possible, choose minimally packaged or package-free goods to help reduce packaging waste and plastic pollution. To eliminate single-use plastics and extra packaging, bring reusable shopping bags, containers, and produce bags.

3. How to conserve energy and resources:

Choose energy-efficient cooking techniques: To save energy and lessen your carbon footprint, choose energy-efficient cooking techniques such as steaming, boiling, or a slow cooker. Choose equipment with excellent energy efficiency ratings and minimize excessive preheating or cooking periods.

Conserve Water: Wash dishes effectively, address leaks quickly, and use water-saving appliances and fixtures. Reduce water waste during food preparation, cooking, and cleaning to help preserve this valuable resource and promote water sustainability.

4. Promoting Ethical and Sustainable Practices:

Select Responsibly Sourced Foods: Choose foods that are produced using ethical and sustainable methods, such as organic, fair trade, and Rainforest Alliance-certified items. Look for eco-friendly certifications and labels that reflect ethical sourcing, environmental stewardship, and fair labor practices.

Advocate for Policy Change: On a local, national, and global scale, advocate for policies and programs that promote sustainable agriculture, environmental conservation, and food system reform. Support organizations and campaigns that advocate for sustainable food production, biodiversity protection, and climate action.

5. Practice mindful consumption:

Embrace Minimalism: Live a minimalist lifestyle by valuing experiences above goods, minimizing needless spending, and simplifying your home. Adopting a minimalist attitude may help you make better-informed decisions, decrease waste, and live more sustainably.

Practice Conscious Consumerism: Make conscious purchase choices by considering environmental effects, ethical issues, and long-term sustainability. Whenever feasible, choose things that are long-lasting, reusable, and created from environmentally friendly materials.

Conclusion:
Intermittent fasting provides a route to better health and well-being, but its advantages might go beyond personal well-being to cover larger environmental sustainability concerns. Individuals who match their fasting habits with sustainable living principles may reduce their environmental impact, promote eco-friendly food systems, and contribute to a healthier world.

As you begin your intermittent fasting adventure, think about the environmental consequences of your food choices, consumption patterns, and lifestyle behaviors. Fasting may be integrated into a sustainable lifestyle that promotes both personal and environmental health by decreasing food waste, selecting sustainable foods, saving energy and resources, supporting ethical actions, and practicing mindful consumption.

Remember that modest adjustments may have a big influence over time, and each decision you make has the potential to contribute to a more sustainable future. By taking a holistic approach to intermittent fasting that considers environmental sustainability, you may feed your body, mind, and planet for long-term health and well-being.

Integrating Intermittent Fasting into Ethical Eating Practices

As concerns about environmental sustainability and ethical food practices develop, many people are looking for methods to connect their eating habits with their beliefs. Intermittent fasting (IF) provides a unique chance to enhance personal health while simultaneously promoting ethical eating and ecological living. In this chapter, we'll look at how intermittent fasting may be integrated into ethical eating practices that promote environmental stewardship, animal welfare, and social responsibility.

Understanding Ethical Food Choices and Intermittent Fasting:

1. Ethical Eating Choices: Ethical eating entails selecting foods that value environmental sustainability, animal welfare, social justice, and ethical food production techniques. Ethical eaters evaluate the influence of their dietary choices on the environment, animals, and communities, aiming to reduce damage while promoting positive change via their food consumption habits.

2. Intermittent Fasting: Intermittent fasting is a kind of eating pattern in which fasting and eating periods alternate. It has gained popularity because of its possible health advantages, which include weight reduction, enhanced metabolic health, and an increased lifespan. Individuals who incorporate intermittent fasting into their diets may improve their health while also aligning their eating choices with ethical and environmental beliefs.

Combining Intermittent Fasting with Ethical Eating Practices:

1. Reduce Meat Consumption:

Prioritize Plant-Based Protein Sources: During meal windows, choose plant-based protein sources such as legumes, tofu, tempeh, nuts, and seeds over animal products. Plant-based proteins have a smaller environmental footprint and help to minimize greenhouse gas emissions, land usage, and water consumption when compared to animal-derived proteins.

Embrace Meatless Meals: Include meatless meals in your fasting days or eating windows to lessen dependency on animal products and promote ethical eating habits. Experiment with vegetarian and vegan dishes that are nutritional, tasty, and enjoyable, highlighting the richness and adaptability of plant-derived ingredients.

2. Support sustainable seafood practices.

Choose sustainable seafood options: To promote ocean health and biodiversity, choose seafood that has been sustainably obtained and harvested. Look for eco-certifications from the Marine Stewardship Council (MSC) or the Aquaculture Stewardship Council (ASC) to verify that seafood products fulfill stringent sustainability criteria.

Decrease Seafood Consumption: Limit seafood consumption to sustainable choices, and decrease total consumption to relieve strain on fragile fish populations and marine ecosystems. Include plant-based alternatives in your diet, such as seaweed, algae, and plant-based seafood replacements, to diversify protein sources and lessen dependency on animal-based proteins.

3. Prioritize organic and local foods.

Pick organic produce: Choose organic fruits and vegetables to promote sustainable agricultural techniques, reduce exposure to pesticides and synthetic chemicals, and maintain soil health and biodiversity. Organic farming practices emphasize soil conservation, water quality, and ecological balance, hence fostering environmental sustainability.

Support Local Farmers: Buy locally produced and seasonal produce at farmers' markets, community-supported agriculture (CSA) programs, or farm-to-table efforts to help local economies, cut food miles, and develop linkages with regional food systems. Supporting local farmers increases agricultural variety, resilience, and food security in your community.

4. Reducing food waste:

Plan Meals Wisely: Plan your meals and fasting schedule carefully to reduce food waste and maximize resource use. Use perishable items before they deteriorate, reuse leftovers imaginatively, and exercise portion control to avoid food waste throughout fasting and feasting times.

Compost food scraps: Use food scraps like fruit and vegetable peels, coffee grinds, and eggshells to divert organic waste from landfills and encourage nutrient cycling in the soil. Composting lowers greenhouse gas emissions, improves soil fertility, and promotes regenerative agricultural methods.

5. Select Ethical Food Brands and Suppliers:

Research Ethical Food Brands: Look for food brands and suppliers that value ethical sourcing, fair labor practices, and supply chain transparency. Look for certifications like Fair Trade, Certified B Corporation, or Animal Welfare. Approved to assist companies that are committed to ethical and sustainable operations.

Vote with Your Money: Show your support for ethical food businesses and products by voting with your money and buying items that reflect your beliefs and ideals. Supporting ethical food producers promotes industry-wide adoption of sustainable and compassionate methods, resulting in positive change in the food system.

6. Educate and advocate.

Raise Awareness: Teach yourself and others about the environmental, social, and ethical consequences of food choices, as well as the advantages of intermittent fasting for personal health and well-being. Share information, ideas, and success stories to encourage others to practice ethical eating and intermittent fasting.

Advocate for Change: Propose legislative changes, industry reforms, and consumer initiatives to promote ethical food production, environmental sustainability, and social justice. Support groups, campaigns, and projects that advocate for food system reform and promote ethical and sustainable food practices at the local, national, and global levels.

Conclusion:

Incorporating intermittent fasting with ethical eating habits helps people improve their health while also promoting environmental sustainability, animal welfare, and social responsibility. Individuals can align their fasting practices with their values by reducing meat consumption, supporting sustainable seafood practices, prioritizing organic and local foods, reducing food waste, selecting ethical food brands and suppliers, and educating and advocating for change.

Remember that every food decision you make has the potential to effect good change and support a healthier, more sustainable future for humans, animals, and the environment. By taking a conscious and purposeful approach to intermittent fasting and ethical eating, you can feed your body, promote ethical food practices, and help to create a more equitable and sustainable world for future generations.

Promoting a Holistic Approach to Health and Wellness

In our pursuit of health and well-being, we must acknowledge that our well-being is inextricably linked to the health of the world and the well-being of all living things. Intermittent fasting (IF), which emphasizes both physical health and sustainable living, offers a unique opportunity to promote a holistic approach to health and well-being. In this chapter, we'll look at how intermittent fasting may be incorporated into a holistic lifestyle that values not just personal health but also environmental sustainability, ethical concerns, and mental and emotional well-being.

Understanding holistic health and wellness.

1. Holistic Health: Holistic health is a multifaceted approach to well-being that considers the interdependence of the body, mind, spirit, and environment. It acknowledges that health is more than just the absence of sickness; it is also a condition of balance and harmony in all areas of life. Holistic health stresses the significance of treating physical, emotional, mental, social, and spiritual elements to attain maximum health.

2. Holistic wellbeing: Holistic wellbeing refers to all aspects of health, including physical, emotional, mental, social, environmental, and spiritual well-being. It focuses on the integration of lifestyle practices, behaviors, and attitudes that promote health, vitality, and satisfaction throughout the life cycle. Holistic wellness acknowledges the link between individual health and the health of the larger community and ecology.

Promoting a Holistic Approach to Health and Wellness via Intermittent Fasting:

1. Physical health:

Improving metabolic health: Intermittent fasting may help regulate blood sugar levels, insulin sensitivity, and lipid profiles.

Fasting may help you maintain metabolic flexibility, burn fat more efficiently, and lower your risk of chronic illnesses, including obesity, type 2 diabetes, and cardiovascular disease.

Promoting Cellular Repair and Renewal: Fasting activates autophagy, a cellular recycling mechanism that eliminates damaged cells and proteins, stimulates cellular repair, and extends life. By fasting regularly, you may help the body's natural cleansing and regeneration processes, increasing cellular health and resilience.

2. Emotional and Mental Wellbeing:

Stress Reduction: Intermittent fasting has been shown to lower stress levels and boost stress resistance by regulating stress response pathways and encouraging neuroplasticity. Fasting causes biochemical changes in the brain that improve mood, cognitive performance, and emotional well-being, resulting in lower anxiety, melancholy, and mood swings.

Improved Cognitive Function: Fasting may improve cognitive function, attention, and mental clarity by increasing the production of brain-derived neurotrophic factor (BDNF) and stimulating neurogenesis. Intermittent fasting improves brain health, memory consolidation, and learning capacity, allowing for peak cognitive performance throughout life.

3. Social Wellbeing:

Community Connection: Intermittent fasting may promote a feeling of belonging and connection via shared experiences, support networks, and online groups. Engaging with people who practice intermittent fasting may provide you with support, encouragement, and companionship on your health path, as well as promote social connections and belonging.

Shared principles: Intermittent fasting is consistent with the principles of mindfulness, simplicity, and sustainability, forging stronger relationships with individuals who share similar values and objectives. By talking about health, wellness, and sustainability, you may form meaningful connections and improve social ties in your community.

4. Environmental Sustainability:

Reduced environmental footprint: Intermittent fasting may help you decrease your environmental impact by encouraging a plant-based diet, avoiding food waste, and conserving resources. Plant-based diets have a smaller carbon footprint, water footprint, and land consumption than animal-based diets, which helps to minimize greenhouse gas emissions and environmental damage.

Promotion of Sustainable Food Systems: Intermittent fasting promotes thoughtful consumption, ethical food choices, and advocacy for sustainable food systems that emphasize environmental stewardship, biodiversity conservation, and social fairness. By incorporating intermittent fasting into your overall lifestyle, you may help to create a more sustainable and resilient food system for future generations.

5. Spiritual and Mindful Practices:

Enhanced Mindfulness: Fasting may strengthen mindfulness techniques by increasing awareness, presence, and attention in everyday life. During fasting times, you may build mindfulness and self-awareness by paying attention to your physiological sensations, thoughts, and emotions, resulting in a stronger connection with yourself and the world around you.

Spiritual Connection: Fasting has long been used for spiritual and religious reasons, promoting a feeling of connection to a greater purpose, inner knowledge, and global awareness. Intermittent fasting may be used as a spiritual practice to feed the soul, enhance faith, and cultivate a feeling of transcendence beyond the physical reality.

Conclusion:

Integrating intermittent fasting into a comprehensive approach to health and well-being may lead to increased energy, balance, and joy. Recognizing the interdependence of body, mind, spirit, and environment, you can build holistic well-being that feeds all areas of your being while also promoting peace with nature.

As you begin your intermittent fasting journey, remember to respect your body's wisdom, prioritize self-care, and acknowledge the interdependence of your health and the health of the earth. By promoting a holistic approach to health and wellbeing via intermittent fasting, you may nurture resilience, energy, and purpose in your life while simultaneously helping to create a more sustainable and compassionate environment for all creatures.

Conclusion

Celebrating Your Journey to Wellness and Vitality

As you near the end of your journey to health and vitality, it's time to stop, reflect, and enjoy your accomplishments, the obstacles you've faced, and the changes you've undergone along the way. Your decision to embrace intermittent fasting as a tool for health and well-being has been a journey of self-discovery, empowerment, and personal development. In closing, let us recognize your accomplishments, praise your perseverance, and celebrate the tremendous influence of your path to well-being and vitality.

Reflecting on your achievements:

1. Personal Development: Throughout your trip, you've been on a road of personal development and self-discovery, discovering your talents, resilience, and inner knowledge. You've shown bravery, drive, and dedication to your well-being by accepting change and venturing outside of your comfort zone in pursuit of a better, more vibrant lifestyle.

2. Health milestones: You've reached key health milestones along the way, including better metabolic health and weight control, as well as increased energy, mental clarity, and emotional well-being. You've personally seen the transformative effect of intermittent fasting on improving your health and vigor, releasing your body's intrinsic healing capacity, and regaining vitality.

3. Lifestyle Changes: Your path has been distinguished by lifestyle and cognitive adjustments that have enabled you to make better decisions and emphasize self-care. You've practiced mindfulness, conscious eating, and holistic well-being, and you've included intermittent fasting as a long-term and empowered lifestyle choice.

Acknowledging Your Resilience

1. Overcoming Challenges: You've had problems, setbacks, and moments of uncertainty along the road, but you've overcome them with tenacity and drive. You've overcome challenges, learned from failures, and adapted to change, exhibiting resilience in the face of adversity while emerging stronger and more resilient as a result.

2. Embracing Growth: Your path has been one of development and evolution, as you've welcomed new experiences, learned from your mistakes, and accepted possibilities for self-improvement. You've embraced change as a catalyst for progress, approaching the unknown with curiosity, openness, and a desire to learn and improve.

3. Cultivating self-compassion: Throughout your journey, you've shown self-compassion, kindness, and self-care, nourishing yourself with love, understanding, and acceptance. You've acknowledged your innate worth and value, and you treat yourself with respect and compassion even when facing a difficulty or setback.

Celebrate Your Journey:

1. Gratitude and Appreciation: Take a minute to express thanks and appreciation for the trip you've made, the lessons you've learned, and the progress you've seen along the way. Celebrate your development, accomplishments, and benefits.

2. Honoring Your Body: Acknowledge and praise your body's resilience, strength, and vitality. Appreciate your body's incredible ability to heal, regenerate, and flourish, and provide it with the care, respect, and appreciation it deserves.

3. Sharing Your Success: Celebrate your triumphs with those who have helped and encouraged you along the way. Celebrate with friends, family, and other wellness lovers, sharing your experiences, thoughts, and achievements to inspire others on their journeys to well-being and vitality.

4. Setting New Goals: As you celebrate your accomplishments, look forward to the future with hope, excitement, and a feeling of possibility. Set new objectives, ambitions, and intentions for your ongoing development and evolution, while welcoming new challenges, chances, and experiences on your path to well-being and vitality.

Conclusion:

As you complete your journey to health and vitality, take pleasure in how far you've come, the challenges you've faced, and the person you've become along the way. Your decision to embrace intermittent fasting as a means of achieving health and well-being demonstrates your bravery, dedication, and perseverance. Celebrate your trip with gratitude, admiration, and delight, knowing that you've set out on a transforming road that has improved your life in innumerable ways.

As you continue your journey, remember to be true to yourself, respect your body, and recognize the value of intermittent fasting as a tool for health, energy, and longevity. Celebrate each step forward, each milestone reached, and each opportunity for development and self-discovery, knowing that you are building a life of health, energy, and purpose.

May your path be blessed with ongoing progress, abundance, and pleasure as you strive for balance, harmony, and well-being. Accept the journey with an open heart, an inquisitive mind, and an adventurous spirit, knowing that the route to well-being and vitality is yours to discover and appreciate every step of the way.

Adopting a Forever Young Mindset with Intermittent Fasting

As we wrap up our investigation of intermittent fasting and its transforming potential for health and well-being, it's time to consider the enormous influence of adopting a "forever young" attitude. Intermittent fasting provides more than simply physical advantages; it also allows you to create a mentality that promotes vigor, resilience, and a young attitude. In this last section, we'll look at the main elements of a "forever young" attitude, how intermittent fasting promotes this thinking, and how to embark on the transforming path of embracing vitality and youthfulness at any age.

Understanding the ever-young mindset:

1. Optimism and Positivity: A perpetually youthful attitude is defined by optimism, enthusiasm, and faith in the possibilities of the future. It entails seeing obstacles as opportunities for growth, being optimistic, and embracing life with a sense of curiosity and wonder.

2) Adaptability and Resilience: Adopting a perpetually youthful attitude requires adaptability and resilience in the face of change and hardship. It entails developing the capacity to recover from setbacks, learn from mistakes, and approach new experiences with an open mind and a desire to learn.

3. Curiosity and lifelong learning: Curiosity, a quest for knowledge, and a dedication to continual learning drive a forever youthful attitude. It entails keeping intellectually active, investigating new ideas and interests, and being open to new opportunities for development and self-discovery.

4. Vitality and Well-Being: The eternally youthful attitude is based on a dedication to vitality and well-being in all parts of life. It entails prioritizing self-care, feeding the body with nutritious food and exercise, and cultivating emotional and mental resilience to promote overall health and vitality.

Intermittent fasting might help you maintain a youthful mindset.

1. Optimizing Health span: Intermittent fasting has been found to improve health span—the amount of time spent free of chronic illness and disability—by boosting cellular repair, lowering inflammation, and improving metabolic function. Intermittent fasting may help your body's natural capacity to heal and regenerate itself, increasing vitality and resilience as you age.

2. Cultivating resilience: Intermittent fasting increases resilience by forcing the body to adjust to times of fasting and feasting. Intermittent fasting stimulates stress response pathways in the body, promoting cellular repair, stress tolerance, and lifespan. Over time, this adaptation enhances the body's capacity to deal with stress and adversity, cultivating a resilient and adaptable attitude.

3. Encouraging interest: Intermittent fasting sparks interest and research by challenging traditional understandings of eating patterns and nutritional habits. As you experiment with various fasting regimens and watch their effects on your body and mind, you develop a feeling of curiosity and wonder about intermittent fasting's potential to improve health and vitality.

4. Promoting Well-Being: Intermittent fasting improves metabolic health, cognitive function, and emotional resilience. Intermittent fasting promotes vigor and well-being by regulating blood sugar levels, improving brain function, and lowering inflammation, generating a feeling of freshness and vibrancy at any age.

The Transformative Journey to Vitality and Youthfulness:

1. Mindset Shift: Embracing a forever youthful attitude is a mindset transformation path that requires a willingness to confront limiting ideas about aging and welcome new possibilities for health and vitality. By redefining your beliefs about aging and accepting the promise of intermittent fasting to promote a vigorous and young lifestyle, you pave the way for revolutionary change.

2. Commitment to Self-Care: Cultivating an eternally youthful attitude includes a dedication to self-care and comprehensive well-being. It involves prioritizing sleep, diet, exercise, and stress management to enhance overall health and vitality. By nourishing your body, mind, and spirit with care and compassion, you establish the basis for a robust and satisfying life.

3. Embracing Change: Adopting a perpetually youthful attitude requires a willingness to welcome change and adjust to new situations with grace and perseverance. It entails letting go of fear, accepting uncertainty, and venturing beyond your comfort zone to achieve progress and self-discovery. By accepting change as a normal aspect of life, you open yourself up to new experiences and opportunities for personal growth.

4. A Celebration of Life: Finally, adopting a forever youthful attitude entails appreciating life in all of its beauty and richness. It's about finding pleasure in the present, being grateful for your blessings, and seeing every day as a chance for development, connection, and adventure. Living with passion, purpose, and excitement for life is the essence of youth at any age.

Conclusion:

As we wrap up our discussion of intermittent fasting and its transforming potential for health and well-being, I ask you to adopt a forever-youthful mindset—an attitude of optimism, resilience, and vigor that allows you to enjoy life to the fullest. By adopting intermittent fasting as a technique for promoting health, vitality, and longevity, you embark on a path of self-discovery and personal change that transcends age and allows you to live life with pleasure, wonder, and enthusiasm.

May your path to energy and youthfulness be blessed with riches, delight and contentment as you develop an attitude of resilience, curiosity, and thankfulness for the great gift of life. Accept the trip with an open heart, an inquisitive mind, and an adventurous spirit, knowing that the path to vitality and youth is yours to discover and cherish every step of the way.

Appendix

Sample Meal Plans and Recipes

In this appendix, we give a variety of example meal plans and dishes to help you on your intermittent fasting journey. Whether you're new to intermittent fasting or seeking new ways to improve your fasting routine, these meal plans and recipes provide tasty and healthy choices to nourish your body, support your health objectives, and make fasting more pleasant. From balanced meals to delectable snacks, these dishes are intended to fit effortlessly into your intermittent fasting regimen while feeding your body and pleasing your taste buds.

Sample meal plans:

1. Meal Plan for 16/8 Intermittent Fasting: Breakfast at 8:00 a.m.

Breakfast Bowl: scrambled eggs, spinach, tomatoes, and avocado over quinoa or brown rice.

Noon (lunch)

Grilled Chicken Salad: mixed greens with grilled chicken breast, cucumber, bell pepper, cherry tomatoes, and balsamic vinaigrette.

Snack at 3:00 PM: Greek Yogurt Parfait with mixed berries, almonds, and honey.

Dinner at 6:00 p.m.

Baked Salmon with Cooked Vegetables: A salmon fillet cooked with Brussels sprouts, carrots, and sweet potatoes.

2. 20/4 Intermittent Fasting Meal Plan: Break Fast at 12:00 PM:

Avocado bread is whole-grain bread with mashed avocado, sliced tomatoes, and a sprinkle of feta cheese.

Lunch at 4:00 PM

Quinoa Salad: Combine quinoa with black beans, corn, sliced bell peppers, cherry tomatoes, cilantro, and lime vinaigrette.

Snack at 6:00 p.m.

Apple with Almond Butter: Sliced apples are served with a dab of almond butter for dipping.

Dinner at 8:00 p.m.

Stir-Fried Tofu with Vegetables: Tofu cooked with broccoli, bell peppers, snap peas, carrots, and a flavorful soy-ginger sauce served over brown rice.

3. Alternate-Day Fasting Meal Plan: Fast Day: 8:00 a.m.

Herbal Tea or Black Coffee: During fasting times, drink a cup of herbal tea or black coffee to aid with appetite and metabolism.

Noon (Fast Day):

Green Salad: A mix of greens, cucumbers, cherry tomatoes, and radishes with a mild vinaigrette dressing.

• 3:00 p.m. (Fast Day):

Veggie Snack Plate: Sliced bell peppers, carrots, celery, and cherry tomatoes served with hummus to dip.

• 6:00 PM (Fast Day):

Vegetable Soup: A homemade soup prepared with onions, garlic, carrots, celery, kale, and vegetable broth.

Sample recipes:

1. Eggs and Vegetable Breakfast Muffins:

Ingredients: 6 eggs.

One cup of chopped veggies (spinach, bell peppers, onions, mushrooms)

1/4 cup shredded cheese.

Add salt and pepper to taste.

- Instructions:

1. Preheat the oven to 350°F/175°C. Coat a muffin tray with cooking spray or line it with paper liners.

2. In a mixing dish, combine the eggs, chopped veggies, shredded cheese, salt, and pepper.

3. Pour the egg mixture into the muffin tray, filling each cup approximately 3/4 full.

4. Bake in the preheated oven for 20–25 minutes, or until the egg muffins are firm and gently browned on top.

5. Let the egg muffins cool slightly before removing them from the muffin tray. Serve it warm or at room temperature.

2. Mediterranean Chickpea Salad:

Ingredients: 1 can (15 oz) of washed and drained chickpeas.

Ingredients: 1 cup halved cherry tomatoes, 1/2 diced English cucumber, and 1/4 finely chopped red onion.

1/4 cup pitted and chopped Kalamata olives.

2 tablespoons fresh parsley, chopped

Ingredients: 2 tablespoons extra virgin olive oil, 1 tablespoon lemon juice.

1 clove garlic, minced

Add salt and pepper to taste.

- Instructions:

1. In a large mixing basin, toss together chickpeas, cherry tomatoes, cucumber, red onion, olives, and parsley.

2. In a small bowl, mix olive oil and lemon juice.

To prepare the dressing, combine minced garlic, salt, and pepper.

3. Pour the dressing over the chickpea mixture and toss to evenly coat.

4. Let the salad marinade for at least 15 minutes before serving so that the flavors may mingle together.

5. Present the Mediterranean chickpea salad as a light and refreshing side dish or main entrée.

3. Coconut Chia Pudding with Fresh Berries:

Ingredients: 1/4 cup chia seeds.

1 cup of coconut milk, either canned or homemade.

Ingredients: 1 tablespoon maple syrup or honey, 1/2 teaspoon vanilla essence.

Topping options include strawberries, blueberries, and raspberries. An optional garnish is shredded coconut.

- Instructions:

1. In a mixing bowl, add the chia seeds, coconut milk, maple syrup (or honey), and vanilla essence.

2. Whisk until fully blended, removing any clumps of chia seeds.

3. Cover the bowl and chill for at least 4 hours, preferably overnight, to enable the chia pudding to thicken and solidify.

4. Before serving, mix the chia pudding well to properly distribute the seeds.

5. Pour the chia pudding into individual serving cups or bowls and garnish with fresh berries and shredded coconut, if preferred.

6. Enjoy the coconut chia pudding as a tasty and healthy dessert or snack.

Resources for Additional Reading and Support

As you continue your intermittent fasting journey, you'll need credible knowledge, support, and tools to help you manage the process efficiently and sustainably. In this appendix, we've assembled a complete list of resources for more reading, research, and support, including books, blogs, podcasts, apps, and online groups focused on intermittent fasting and related subjects. Whether you want to learn more about intermittent fasting, find inspiration and motivation, or connect with like-minded people, these sites provide vital insights, information, and encouragement to help you on your health path.

Books:

1. Dr. Jason Fung's "The Obesity Code" In this ground-breaking book, Dr. Jason Fung investigates the root causes of obesity and presents the notion of intermittent fasting as a potent tool for weight reduction and metabolic health. Dr. Fung, drawing on scientific research and clinical expertise, offers practical advice on how to apply intermittent fasting for long-term outcomes.

2) "The Complete Guide to Fasting" by Dr. Jason Fung and Jimmy Moore: This thorough resource provides a plethora of information about intermittent fasting, including its advantages, various fasting regimens, and practical success strategies. Dr. Fung and co-author Jimmy Moore's ideas will help readers develop a better grasp of how fasting may improve health and well-being.

3. "Delay, Don't Deny" by Gin Stephens: In this fascinating and relevant book, intermittent fasting advocate Gin Stephens describes her own fasting experience and provides practical tips for bringing fasting into daily life. "Delay, Don't Deny" encourages readers to adopt a long-term approach to intermittent fasting by emphasizing flexibility, mindfulness, and self-discovery.

Websites:

1. The Obesity Code Site (https://theobesitycode.com/): Dr. Jason Fung's website has a plethora of information on intermittent fasting, including articles, videos, and success stories from people who have benefitted from it. Visitors may get free materials, participate in online forums, and learn more about Dr. Fung's approach to fasting and metabolic health.

2. The Intensive Dietary Management website (https://idmprogram.com/): Dr. Jason Fung and Megan Ramos founded the Intensive Dietary Management (IDM) program, which provides tailored coaching and support to anyone interested in fasting for weight reduction and metabolic health. The website includes instructional information, success stories, and online courses to assist people in achieving their health objectives.

3. The Delay, Don't Deny Community (https://www.dontdeny.com/) Gin Stephens' online community allows people who practice intermittent fasting to interact, share their experiences, and seek advice from experienced fasters. Members may access forums, take part in group challenges, and discover inspiration to keep them inspired throughout their fasting journey.

Podcasts:

1. Intermittent Fasting Podcast: This popular podcast, hosted by Gin Stephens and Melanie Avalon, delves into all elements of intermittent fasting, including varied fasting regimens and practical success strategies. With informative interviews, Q&A sessions, and real-life success stories, the program provides important support and motivation to listeners.

2) The Obesity Code Podcast: Dr. Jason Fung conducts this podcast, which covers the most recent research and insights into obesity, metabolic health, and the advantages of intermittent fasting. Listeners may benefit from Dr. Fung's knowledge and practical recommendations for incorporating fasting into their lifestyle.

3. Life Omic Podcast: Fasting Talk: This podcast, hosted by Dr. Jason Fung and Megan Ramos, explores the science of fasting and its possible influence on health and lifespan. The podcast provides vital information and support to those interested in fasting through in-depth talks, professional interviews, and listener Q&A sessions.

Apps:

1. Zero: Zero is fasting tracker software that enables users to measure their progress, set goals, and see their fasting history. Zero's configurable fasting clocks, educational materials, and community support help users stay inspired and accountable throughout their fasting journey.

2. Life fasting Tracker: Life is a complete fasting app that supports a variety of fasting regimens, including 16/8, 18/6, OMAD (One Meal a Day), and prolonged fasts. Users may keep track of their fasting hours, record their meals, and interact with a supportive network of other fasts for encouragement and inspiration.

3. MyFitnessPal: While not intended for fasting, MyFitnessPal is a popular software for monitoring food consumption, exercise, and weight reduction progress. Users may record their meals, manage macronutrients, and monitor their calorie intake to help them achieve their intermittent fasting objectives.

Online communities:

1. The Reddit Intermittent Fasting Community (r/intermittent fasting): With over 1.5 million members, this dynamic online community allows people to share their stories, ask questions, and seek help with their intermittent fasting journey. Members may engage in conversations, exchange success stories, and get incentives to stick to their fasting objectives.

2. Facebook Intermittent Fasting Groups: There are various Facebook groups devoted to intermittent fasting, covering a wide range of fasting regimens, food preferences, and health aims. These communities provide a friendly atmosphere in

which members may interact, exchange information, and encourage one another on their fasting journeys.

3. Instagram Intermittent Fasting Community: Instagram has a thriving community of intermittent fasting aficionados who post their fasting experience, food ideas, and progress images with hashtags like intermittent fasting, fasting life, and fasting journey. Users who follow accounts devoted to intermittent fasting might get inspiration, suggestions, and encouragement to keep on track with their fasting objectives.

Conclusion:

Remember that you are not alone on your intermittent fasting adventure. With a multitude of resources for further reading, research, and support, you'll have access to a community of experts, other fasters, and essential knowledge to help you along the road. Whether you're looking for books to help you understand fasting, websites to access educational materials, podcasts to listen to on the go, apps to track your progress, or online communities to connect with like-minded people, intermittent fasting can help you learn, grow, and thrive. Accept the trip with curiosity, openness, and dedication to your health and well-being, knowing you have the information, resources, and support you need to succeed on your fasting adventure.

Glossary

Intermittent fasting (IF) is a dietary pattern in which one fasts and then eats. It does not dictate which foods to consume or avoid, but rather when to eat them.

Fasting window: the time during which one refrains from ingesting food or caloric drinks. It might last from a few hours to a whole day or more, depending on the fasting strategy.

Feeding window: the period within which all meals and caloric drinks are consumed when intermittent fasting. It often occurs during the fasting window and might vary in length based on the fasting procedure.

Autophagy is a cellular process that breaks down and recycles damaged or defective components to promote cellular repair and regeneration. Autophagy is thought to be stimulated during fasting.

Ketosis is a metabolic state in which the body predominantly uses fat for fuel rather than carbs. Ketosis is usually established during times of fasting or reduced carbohydrate consumption.

Insulin resistance is a disorder in which cells become less sensitive to insulin, resulting in high blood sugar levels. Insulin resistance is a typical precursor to type 2 diabetes, and it is often related to obesity and metabolic syndrome.

Metabolic syndrome is a group of diseases that include obesity, high blood pressure, raised blood sugar levels, and abnormal lipid levels, all of which raise the risk of heart disease, stroke, and type 2 diabetes.

Adipose tissue is body fat that stores extra energy in the form of triglycerides. Adipose tissue controls energy balance and metabolic wellness.

Glucose is a basic sugar that cells use as their major source of energy. The breakdown of carbohydrates in the diet produces glucose, which is then carried into the circulation to power cellular operations.

Glycogen is a complex carbohydrate found in the liver and muscles that serve as a reserve energy source. When blood sugar levels drop, glycogen is converted into glucose, providing a quick source of energy during fasting or exercise.

Ghrelin is a hormone generated by the stomach that stimulates appetite and increases food intake. Ghrelin levels normally increase before and fall after meals.

Leptin is a hormone generated by fat cells that affect hunger and energy levels. When fat reserves are adequate, leptin tells the brain to eat less and burn more calories.

Calorie restriction (CR) is a dietary intervention that reduces calorie intake while avoiding malnutrition. In many animal models, calorie restriction has been demonstrated to increase longevity and enhance metabolic health.

Metabolic rate: the pace at which the body expends energy to maintain essential physiological activities, including breathing, circulation, and digestion. Age, body composition, and degree of exercise all have an impact on metabolic rate.

Body mass index (BMI) is a measurement of body fat based on height and weight, computed by dividing weight in kilograms by height in meters squared. BMI is used to divide people into four categories: underweight, normal weight, overweight, and obese.

Lean body mass (LBM) is the body's total weight minus body fat. Lean body mass is made up of muscle, bone, organs, and other non-fat structures.

Satiety is the sense of fullness and contentment that comes after eating a meal. Meal composition, portion size, and eating pace all have an impact on satiety.

Hormesis is a biological phenomenon in which low amounts of stress or toxins trigger adaptive responses that increase resistance and lifespan. Exercising, fasting, and being exposed to cold or heat are examples of hormonal stresses.

Circadian rhythm is the natural internal clock that governs sleep-wake cycles, hormone release, and other physiological functions during 24 hours. Light and temperature are examples of environmental signals that regulate circadian rhythms.

Fasting mimicking diet (FMD): a dietary regimen that mimics the effects of fasting while allowing for some food consumption. FMD is often achieved by following a low-calorie, plant-based diet for a certain length of time.

Thermogenesis is the process by which the body creates heat to maintain its temperature. Thermogenesis may increase during fasting or activity because the body burns calories for energy.

Hypoglycemia refers to abnormally low blood sugar levels, which may cause symptoms such as weakness, dizziness, sweating, and disorientation. Hypoglycemia may result from extended fasting or as a side effect of some drugs.

Electrolytes: minerals such as sodium, potassium, and magnesium that transport electrical charges and play critical roles in fluid equilibrium, neuron function, and muscle contraction. Electrolyte imbalances may develop during fasting or dehydration, resulting in symptoms such as weakness, cramps, and an irregular heartbeat.

Fasting insulin refers to the amount of insulin in the blood during fasting periods, which indicates insulin sensitivity and general metabolic health. Fasting insulin levels are usually lower in those with normal metabolic function.

Omega-3 fatty acids are polyunsaturated fats found in fatty fish, flaxseed, chia seeds, and walnuts. Omega-3 fatty acids have anti-inflammatory effects and are beneficial to heart health, cognitive function, and general well-being.

Oxidative stress is a condition defined by an imbalance between free radicals and antioxidants in the body, resulting in cellular damage and inflammation. Oxidative stress is linked to aging, chronic illness, and degenerative disorders.

Telomeres are protective caps on the ends of chromosomes that serve to maintain chromosomal integrity and prevent DNA damage. Telomeres shorten with age and are considered a sign of cellular aging and longevity.

Neurogenesis is the process by which new neurons are formed in the brain, particularly in the hippocampus and other areas related to learning and memory. Exercise, fasting, and cognitive stimulation may all promote neurogenesis.

Mitochondria are organelles inside cells that generate energy in the form of adenosine triphosphate (ATP) via oxidative phosphorylation. Mitochondria are crucial for cellular metabolism, energy generation, and general health.

Index

A
- Adipose tissue
- Alternate-Day Fasting
- Anti-aging effects
- Appetite regulation
- Autophagy

B
- BMI (Body Mass Index)
- Blood sugar regulation
- Books on intermittent fasting

C
- Calorie restriction
- Circadian rhythm
- Cognitive function
- Community support
- Cooking tips
- Cortisol
- Creativity

D
- Delay, Don't Deny (DDD)
- Diabetes prevention
- Dietary patterns
- Digestive health
- Dopamine

E
- Eating window
- Electrolytes
- Emotional eating
- Energy levels
- Environmental sustainability
- Exercise benefits
- Extended fasting

F
- Fat loss
- Fasting mimicking diet (FMD)
- Feeding window
- Fiber intake
- Flexibility
- Food cravings
- Food diary
- Food quality
- Free radicals

G
- Ghrelin
- Glycogen
- Gut microbiome

H
- Health span
- Heart health
- Herbal teas
- Hormesis
- Hormonal balance
- Hunger cues
- Hydration

I
- IF (Intermittent Fasting)
- Insulin resistance
- Insulin sensitivity

K
- Ketosis

L
- Lean body mass
- Leptin
- Lifestyle changes
- Longevity
- Low-carb diets

M
- Macronutrients
- Meal planning
- Metabolic rate
- Metabolic syndrome
- Mindful eating
- Mitochondria
- Mood regulation
- Motivation

N
- Neurogenesis
- Nutrient density
- Nutritional supplements

O
- Omega-3 fatty acids
- Optimal health
- Overeating

P
- Plateaus
- Podcasts on intermittent fasting
- Portion control
- Protein intake

Q
- Quality sleep

R
- Recipes
- Reducing inflammation
- Resilience
- Resources for further reading
- Restrictive eating patterns

S
- Satiety
- Self-awareness
- Self-care
- Social support
- Stress management
- Sustainable living

T
- Telomeres
- Time-restricted feeding
- Thermogenesis
- Tools for tracking progress

U
- Understanding hunger cues

V
- Vegan diets
- Vegetarian diets
- Vitality
- Vitamins and minerals

W
- Water fasting
- Weight loss
- Whole foods